Dynamic Psychotherapy Explained

PATRIC
Senio
Depar
St Ge

RADC

Radcliffe Medical Press Ltd
18 Marcham Road, Abingdon, Oxon OX14 1AA

British Library Cataloguing in Publication Data

A catalogue record for this book is available from the British Library.

ISBN 1 85775 336 4

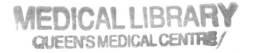
Typeset by Advance Typesetting Ltd, Oxfordshire
Printed and bound by Biddles Ltd, Guildford and King's Lynn

Contents

About the author

Patricia Hughes MBChB, MSc, FRCPsych is Senior Lecturer and Consultant in Psychotherapy at St George's Hospital Medical School and Pathfinder Mental Health Trust in London. She is an Associate Member of the British Psychoanalytical Society and a Group Analyst.

Preface

This book is intended for beginners in psychiatry including postgraduate trainees in psychiatry, psychiatric nursing and general practice, and undergraduate medical and nursing students. I have tried to give a clear and simple outline of the theory and practice of dynamic psychotherapy. As the book is primarily intended for students whose interest and training is predominantly biological, the theory has been put into the context of a model of mental functioning which integrates a biological and a psychological approach.

Chapter 1 gives an outline of the neurobiology of emotion and of the nature of mental representation, with particular reference to the interaction of genes and environment in the development of the brain, and the implications for mental processes. Chapter 2 explains where psychotherapy lies in relation to models of the mind and brain which underlie the theory and practice of general psychiatry. Chapter 3 describes the place of dynamic psychotherapy in relation to other commonly practised psychotherapies. Chapter 4 outlines the theory and Chapter 5 the practice of psychodynamic psychotherapy.

Both undergraduates and postgraduate trainees have a huge amount to read and learn and this is intended to be a text that can be read rapidly and easily grasped. This has inevitably led to oversimplification of complex concepts. There are well-written books which give a full account of theory and practice and interested students and intending specialists should read them. References within the text are given in full at the end of each chapter, with suggestions for further reading related to the material of the chapter.

At the end of the book there is a list of texts which I have found particularly useful.

When I was a medical student 30 years ago I thought that psychotherapy was a fascinating area, but had only the vaguest understanding of the theory behind it, and an ill-formulated notion of what kind of people might benefit and how psychotherapy was practised. Even as a trainee beginning psychiatry, although good textbooks were available I found the level of explanation was often beyond me. I realise that I have written the book which I would have liked to have had then, and I hope it may help the next generation of students and trainees in both psychiatry and nursing to understand and enjoy an important area of psychiatry.

The book was written with NHS clinicians in mind, and I have used the convention of calling people who have therapy 'patients'. Therapists and patients may be female or male, but the use of 'he or she' is clumsy and impedes easy reading. Where either could be used, I have used 'she' for the therapist, and have used 'he' for everyone else.

Patricia Hughes
December 1998

Acknowledgements

I should like to thank Gerald Wooster for engaging my interest in psychoanalysis nearly 20 years ago, Janet Boakes, Sarah Robertson, Daniel Fordwour, John Stevens, Susan Davison and Marina Perris, who have been stimulating and supportive colleagues for many years, and Arthur Crisp, who encouraged the staff of his department at St George's Hospital Medical School to take teaching seriously. I would not have returned to reading neurobiology without the stimulus of Mark Solms' illuminating seminars on psychoanalysis and the brain, and would have been lost without Robert Lawrence's clear explanations. Helen Bond, Susan Davison, Jim Bolton and Marco Piccioni are busy clinicians who generously read drafts of the text and whose suggestions have been immensely helpful. As usual I have had patient support from George Hughes who has willingly read and reread drafts of the book, and given unstinting encouragement.

In memory of Marion Burgner

Introduction

Treatments for mental disorders are as old as the recorded history of medicine, and probably older. Interventions of various kinds have been documented for centuries, but like treatments of physical illnesses were restricted by a limited understanding of the structure and organisation of body and mind. Most early interventions were based either on magical ideas of manipulating the mind or on physical restraint, sometimes cruelly applied and well documented, for example in the history of the Bethlem Hospital in London.

In the past 50 years the enormous strides made in developing effective drug treatments and improvements in diagnostic instruments have given us potent tools to improve mental symptoms by chemical means. As a result, people with some of the most serious mental illnesses can now have hope of remission, and sometimes recovery, which would not have been possible 50 years ago. But despite their value to some patients, chemical treatments have not proved able to help all people with mental disorder. There is an important place for psychological treatments, either as an alternative or in combination with drug therapy.

The ideas of Sigmund Freud in the early part of the 20th century were a powerful influence in developing psychological interventions based on a coherent model of the mind. The fact that Freud the psychoanalyst was also a doctor and a specialist in neuroscience led him to develop theories that were consistent with what was then known about the ways in which the brain functions. This link with biological knowledge remains important for the place of psycho-dynamic psychotherapy in medical practice.

Clinical practice has changed since Freud's day. Psychoanalysis can only ever be available to relatively few people, and the original technique has been modified to offer shorter and less intensive treatments to the many people who seek psychotherapy. Interest in particular problems has stimulated study of specific interventions, for example for people with borderline personality disorder. The recent emphasis on evidence-based practice in medicine has been a further spur to evaluate existing methods and to defining effective techniques.

Further reading

Ellenberger HF (1970) *The Discovery of the Unconscious: the history and evolution of dynamic psychiatry*. Basic Books, New York.

Porter R (1996) *Cambridge Illustrated History of Medicine*. Cambridge University Press, Cambridge.

A developmental model of the mind

Brain and mind • The mind–brain relationship • Born or made: the nature–nurture debate • The neurobiology of emotion • The effect of experience on the developing brain • The effect of severe deprivation on the developing brain • The effect of experience on the mature brain • The nature of mental representations • Mental representations and relating to the world

Brain and mind

MAIN POINTS

- The brain contains the representation of experience which makes a person an individual.

- *Mind* is the word used to designate the 'higher functions of the brain', namely thinking and feeling.

- From birth, human infants organise experience on the basis of similarities and differences. Experience is stored in the brain as

continued …

neurally encoded mental representations of self and other with an associated affect.

- Mental representations have multiple associations to other thoughts and memories. Many associations are determined by social and cultural rules rather than by anatomical ones. These associations give meaning to a person's thoughts, feelings and behaviour.

- This level of organisation constitutes *psychological* organisation.

The brain as a special organ

The brain is the only one of our organs which could not conceivably be given to another person. It is special because it changes so much from birth to childhood to adult life, and changes in a particular way. All my experience, all the interactions of my body with the environment, are registered in the brain. And these experiences and the thoughts, memories and dreams which they stimulate make me the individual I am. I could not even give my brain to my own child or my identical twin. The transplant would be the rest of the body, because the brain contains whatever it is that makes me me. If this is taken away then I am effectively dead.

The functions of the brain

The functions of the brain include:

- sensory perception
- movement and motor control
- autonomic control
- the so-called 'higher' functions of thinking and feeling.

What do we mean by the mind?

The term 'mind' is used to designate the higher functions of the brain. The human brain or mind is different from the computer brain because it is linked to a body through which we experience the world. Mature functioning in the adult human brain requires that the brain has made representations of experience. These include the vast range of sensory, motor and interpersonal experiences which take place from infancy onwards.

Development of the mind

Developmental studies show that as the child acquires experiences, it classifies them according to similarities and differences. These are across a range of variables including physical characteristics, associated thoughts, emotional content and innumerable combinations of these. The representation in the brain is widespread, with a huge number of synaptic connections and not localised in one particular area. These representations of experience give meaning to a person's thoughts and behaviours. This is a new level of organisation in the brain, the level of organisation according to meaning and association.

Thus we have anatomical organisation, physiological organisation and psychological organisation. For the most part a person shares anatomical and physiological organisation with the species, but psychological organisation, although having much in common with other people, is also individual.

Psychological organisation

Mental representations have multiple associative links to other representations. As experience accumulates, the range of associations which determine how it is organised increases exponentially. Many of the associations are determined by social and cultural rules rather than primarily biological ones.

Thus a great deal of mental content is organised in terms of its meaning for the person. This is how we access it in psychotherapy – by understanding or attempting to understand the rules which the individual uses to represent self and the world. We assume that mental process and mental representations have a biological substrate, i.e. that thoughts for example do not take place without activity at a synaptic level. Whether thoughts are the same thing as synaptic activity is the subject of much philosophical debate (*see* Solms, 1997).

The mind–brain relationship

MAIN POINTS

- Change in the physical or chemical structure of the brain leads to mental change.

- Change in mental activity such as learning leads to change in brain structure.

- Much psychological organisation is complex and does not correspond with discrete anatomical areas.

- Evaluating mental representation will be a more useful way to access a person's psychological working model of the world than exploring anatomical or physiological organisation.

The brain is the organ of the mind and mental events must correspond to neurobiological activity in the brain. We assume that mental activities (for example, thought and feeling, memory, belief and desire) are accompanied by brain activity, chemical, electrical and structural. This does not necessarily tell us that the one is caused by the other, although we know that the activities of brain and mind impinge each on the other. This is important when critically evaluating articles, especially in the popular press where there is a common misunderstanding between *correlation* and *cause*.

Change in the physical or chemical structure of the brain leads to psychological change, and psychological experience leads to anatomical and physiological change. For example, experiments with drugs show that chemicals can change mental state, and diseases, such as brain tumours which affect brain structure, can cause changes in mental functioning. Research on immature (infant), non-human primates has shown that environmental modification leads to differences in both anatomical structure and chemical function in the brain (Kraemer, 1992). Experiments on adult animals demonstrate that new learning leads to changes in the structure of the brain (Kandel *et al.*, 1995). Recent work with neuroimaging has shown that some brain activity corresponding to mental activity can be observed in visual representations of the brain.

The anatomical structure of the brain can be identified either macroscopically by dissection of the brain, or using radiographic techniques which provide images of the living and active brain. We can directly link some mental activity, for example visual perception, to anatomical areas of the brain. With assays of fluids and tissues in the brain and nervous system we can discover the physiological processes that operate within the brain, and we know, for example, that when we are emotionally aroused there will be a change in the level of biogenic amines in the central nervous system.

There are particular areas of the brain whose integrity is essential for certain aspects of psychological functioning. For example, if a person suffers severe injury to the prefrontal cortex, then the capacity to regulate emotional arousal will be lost and the person will show emotional outbursts and disinhibited behaviour.

However, an understanding of anatomy and physiology cannot fully explain complex behaviours like the ability to make friends, to work effectively or to feel self-confident. To make sense of these we need to investigate the psychological representations of self and the world which organise our behaviour. These mental representations will be the end result of interaction between genetic inheritance, social or environmental experience and the current life situation.

Born or made: the nature–nurture debate

MAIN POINTS

- Gene expression depends to an extent on environmental influences.

- Early environmental events are likely to have long-lasting effect on the immature organism.

- Behaviour, thoughts and feelings emerge as a result of the interaction of the genetic potential of the individual and the environment.

- Our knowledge of the genetic heritability of most psychological disorders is limited, so our ideas about heritability are rather speculative.

continued ...

- A few diseases are entirely genetically determined. Most have both an environmental and a genetic component. With many we do not know the relative contribution of genes and environment.

- Even disorders which are mainly determined by the impact of the environment must have a biological, though not necessarily a genetic, component.

- Changes brought about by social or psychotherapeutic intervention must ultimately affect the organism at the level of connections between synapses.

Genes that programme the development of biological and psychological structures begin their effect before birth. The activation of the potential effect of a gene is called 'expression of the gene'. Some genes are inevitably expressed regardless of the environment in which the person is living. Others will be expressed to a greater or lesser extent depending on what happens to the organism (person), especially while it is immature. The principle that early events of development have long-lasting effects is one of the elemental precepts shared by all disciplines which study living organisms. The environment begins to exert its influence *in utero* and becomes of prime importance after birth.

We inherit DNA from our biological parents. Behaviour, thoughts and feelings are not inherited. They are the outcome of the interaction of environment on our inherited genes. Another way of thinking about this is to say that behaviour, thoughts and feelings emerge as a result of the impact of environmental factors on the developing neural circuitry.

Studies of identical twins reared apart reveal similarities in attitude and personality and indicate that human behaviour has a significant hereditary component. Further evidence is seen in the ability to select and breed behavioural traits in laboratory and domestic animals. However, even identical twins reared together do not experience identical environmental conditions, and despite their similarities, do show distinct differences in personality.

Some mental diseases are entirely genetically determined, such as Huntington's chorea. If one identical twin has the disease, the other will inevitably be affected. Other diseases are only partly genetically determined. Schizophrenia is considered to have a genetic component in its multifactorial aetiology. If one identical twin develops schizophrenia, his twin has a 40% chance of getting the disease compared with a 10% risk for non-identical twins. Thus we can see that schizophrenia is a disease in which both genetic and environmental factors play a part.

For many years psychiatry was dominated by a debate about whether mental illness is caused by biological or psychosocial factors. This is an unhelpful way to conceptualise the causes of mental illness. A more useful question might be 'How do biological processes in the brain give rise to mental events, and how do social factors modify the biological structure of the brain?' A balanced clinical approach will consider to what degree a mental disorder is determined by genetic factors, to what degree by developmental and environmental factors, and to what degree it is socially defined.

Even disorders that are heavily determined by social or developmental factors must have a biological aspect, because it is the activity of the brain that is being modified. In so far as psychosocial intervention works, whether it is psychotherapy or social manipulation of the environment, it must ultimately impinge on the individual by changing the connections between nerve cells. The absence of demonstrable structural change does not mean that change has not occurred. The currently available technology simply does not allow assessment or evaluation of biological change at a synaptic level.

The neurobiology of emotion

MAIN POINTS

- Our external perceptions are mediated by the sensory modalities.
- Awareness of our internal state may be considered an internal perception.

continued ...

- Arousal is physiological response to perception which prepares the body for action.

- Thinking is a complex activity involving many areas of the brain but predominantly the association areas of the cortex.

- Emotion is different from arousal because it is a meaningful mental state, made so by associated thoughts and memories.

- Drugs which act on the mind do so by affecting the neuronal circuits which mediate emotional arousal.

Jane goes to her car after work and finds that the window has been smashed and realises that her car has been broken into. She feels anxious and angry, she feels her pulse racing and remembers that there has been a spate of car thefts recently. She decides that the sensible thing to do is to see what has been stolen and report the matter to the police.

Jane has a perception (sensory system) of the broken window. This triggers thoughts with associated memories and feelings (higher cortical functions). These lead in turn to somatic responses (autonomic system). On the basis of the information now available to the brain, Jane plans a response to the perception (higher function), which includes motor action (motor activity). Thus, the sensory, autonomic, motor and 'higher' functions of the brain are intricately connected.

The nature of perception

External perceptions are mediated by the sensory modalities: vision, hearing, somatic sensation, taste and smell. Each of these combines different modalities. For example, somatic sensation combines: touch, pain, temperature, vibration, joint sense and muscle sense.

The so-called properties of the physical world are defined by the perceptual properties of the human brain. If none of us could see, then we should conceive of the objects in the external world in quite a different way from our present conception as seeing beings. And if a creature from another planet arrived with a sensory capacity in a new modality, then new properties of the outside world would emerge. Intriguingly, this also applies to our own bodies. We can only know them with the sensory apparatus available to us.

A person's awareness of his or her own emotional or feeling state may be considered to be an internal perception. Just as we have a visual cortex, an auditory cortex and so on for the external sensory modalities, so do we have an affective cortex which allows conscious recognition of feeling states.

Arousal

Physiological responses to perceptions are part of the autonomic system of the body, are generally outside conscious control and prepare the body for action. These are designated as states of arousal. Arousal occurs when, for example, we are joyful, when we laugh or cry, are surprised, frightened or angry. The components of arousal are variations in motor activity, including changes in heart rate and peripheral circulation, and electrophysiological correlates, including sweating and skin conduction changes. The pattern of arousal associated with each emotion is different although there is a good deal of overlap between, for example, pleasurable excitement and fear.

Unlike emotion, arousal does not have specific meaning for the person. When we experience the signs of physical arousal without being able to identify the reason, we tend to feel fear, assuming something is wrong with our body. We can produce states of meaningless arousal by artificially stimulating parts of the brain. Thus a person can experience rage and all its associated bodily responses following stimulation of the medial part of the amygdala, but the rage will be without meaning for the subject.

Thinking

Cognition or thinking does not take place in one area of the brain, but certain areas are more concerned with thinking than others. The association areas of the brain are concerned with integration of somatic information with other sensory modalities, with emotional behaviour, memory, language and the planning of movement.

There are three major association areas in the cortex:

- prefrontal
- parietal-temporal-occipital
- limbic.

Each association area is specialised in function, though all three contribute to more than one cognitive function.

Prefrontal association cortex

The prefrontal area is a large area at the anterior end of the frontal cortex. It is important for weighing the consequences of future actions and planning accordingly.

Parietal-temporal-occipital association cortex

This area is important in processing sensory information for perception and language, and thus for learning spatial tasks and for knowledge of the body in space, i.e. body image.

Limbic association cortex

This area includes the orbitofrontal cortex (which is actually part of the prefrontal cortex), cingulate region and parahippocampal area. The limbic association cortex allows emotions to affect motor planning.

Although the integrity of the association areas is essential for a person's effective functioning, thinking cannot be simply localised to these areas. Thinking is an immensely complex process, involving thousands of neuronal links with different areas of the brain, and to an extent different areas of the brain can compensate for loss in another area. When a part of the brain is removed experimentally, the behaviour of the animal afterwards may be as much a reflection of the adjusted capacity of the remaining brain as of the function of the part of the brain that was removed.

Emotions (also called *affects*)

Emotion is the perception of an inner state, which includes a perception of: (i) level and quality of arousal; (ii) degrees of pleasure and/ or displeasure (discomfort); and (iii) associated thoughts. Emotions are always accompanied by thoughts, and thoughts by emotions. Sometimes neither the thoughts nor somatic changes which accompany an emotion fully reach conscious awareness.

Except in laboratory settings, where there may be direct brain stimulation, emotions and states of arousal are stimulated by external perceptions and by memories and thoughts. In certain brain diseases, a person may suffer from apparently inexplicable states of arousal triggered by brain dysfunction.

The autonomic, endocrine and skeletomotor responses which accompany arousal, and therefore emotion, depend on subcortical structures. These include the amygdala, hypothalamus and brainstem. The hippocampus is important for memory and plays a role in linking current perception with the relevant emotional state.

The emotional response of an individual to any situation is influenced by the *personal meaning* of what is perceived. Personal meaning of a perception is largely defined by present context and by the person's mental representations of previous experiences and the memories and associations to these. Emotion becomes meaningful largely because of the activities of the cortex, and especially the association cortex. Emotions are not always fully conscious, and there are many reasons why a particular emotion is kept out of conscious awareness. This may be important in clinical practice.

Many drugs that act on the mind (including both street drugs and therapeutic drugs) exert their action by affecting the neuronal circuits which mediate the physiological component of emotions. These drugs affect level of arousal and/or degree of pleasure. Such states of pleasurable arousal are chemically generated and not meaningful in any personal sense.

The effect of experience on the developing brain

MAIN POINTS

- The infant brain is immature at birth. It has most of its neurones (brain cells), but relatively few synapses (connections).

- The prefrontal cortex, and particularly the orbitofrontal part of the prefrontal cortex, is the part of the brain that controls emotional regulation and verbal learning.

- In the first two years, there is an overproduction of synapses in the prefrontal cortex which is then thinned down by selection of the connections which are most used. Unused connections die.

- Prefrontal development is driven by environmental stimulation.

- Environmental experience in the early years determines the connections in the cortex which are established at that time.

- The presence of an interested care-giver in the first two years is important for the development of the ability to relate to other people. This includes among other things the use of language, capacity for empathy and the regulation of emotion.

Complex functional brain systems are not ready-made at birth. They are formed during the processes of sensory stimulation, social contact and interactive activity by the child. The infant develops connections between synapses depending on how much they are used.

An infant has to have certain environmental conditions for healthy brain and mind development. We cannot simply keep the baby warm, clean and fed and expect that the brain and mental function will develop spontaneously.

During the first few years of life the brain of the human child goes through stages of intense activity (critical periods) when numerous lines of communication are set up. These critical periods of cortical development are highly dependent on experience, i.e. stimulation from the environment. The process continues throughout life, but the pace is far slower in the adult brain.

The child's earliest social relationship with the environment, of which the mother (or primary care-giver) is a large and important part, will to an extent determine the child's subsequent approach to relating to the external world. Early experiences influence the development of neural pathways which are the biological substrate of the personality, its adaptive capacities and strengths, and its vulnerabilities to particular forms of future pathology. Thus the emergence of a healthy personality requires more than the inborn ability to organise experience. It also needs the presence of others who provide certain types of experience.

The postnatally developing prefrontal cortex is the part of the brain that inhibits drive and regulates arousal. Healthy development in this part of the brain more than any other needs the presence of others who offer adequate and appropriate emotional and cognitive experience (Schore, 1994).

Repeated early emotional interactions with the social environment are mentally stored in the form of representations of the self interacting with a significant other and a linking, mediating emotion. These representations are a configuration of thoughts and feelings which have social meaning, but they are also neuronal. Thus social and psychological experience is internalised as a permanent and individual modification of the nervous system.

Clinically, we will not make much progress trying to understand the rules governing how these representations are organised anatomically because the neuronal connections are so widespread and so numerous (there are 10^{14} neuronal connections in the adult human brain), and because many of the connections are specific to the individual. We are more likely to get an understanding of the way a person's mind works by accessing the groups of representations of relationships in the way in which they were laid down, i.e. by studying the relationship between behaviour, thoughts and feelings, sometimes in a psychosocial setting or therapeutic relationship.

The effect of severe deprivation on the developing brain

MAIN POINTS

- Work has been done on non-human primates which suggests that severe deprivation has a profound effect on the immature central nervous system.

- Infant monkeys who experience prolonged isolation in infancy have lower levels of CNS noradrenaline (norepinephrine) and thinning of the dendritic branching in the cortex and cerebellum. They have post-synaptic hypersensitivity to noradrenaline leading to overreaction to stress.

- They show severe behavioural abnormalities including 'isolation syndrome' and despair response to later separation.

- Rehabilitation is difficult. Care from 'therapist' peers is most successful. This improves social behaviour but does not help the CNS abnormalities.

- Even after rehabilitation the monkeys lack the ability to deal with stress and may become lethally aggressive.

- This raises the question of how a person who has been severely deprived in early childhood can best be helped with psycho-social difficulties later in life.

One way in which we can research the development of the brain is to examine what happens when an immature brain is deprived of the usual stimulation. We cannot ethically experiment with rearing human infants under conditions of severe social deprivation but such experiments have been done with non-human primates. Studies of severely deprived monkey infants have explored which aspects of the mother are essential for normal behavioural and normal central nervous system (CNS) development to take place. If the infant monkey is removed from the mother, neither soft dummy surrogates, rocking surrogates nor alternative animal surrogates achieve full normality for the monkey's development. It must be concluded that the mother has specific characteristics which make her the best caretaker of the infant monkey.

If infant monkeys are separated from the mother from birth to six months, cerebrospinal fluid (CSF) noradrenaline (norepinephrine) is markedly lower than in mother-reared monkeys and does not return to normal even if the monkeys are then returned to the group. There is also a reduction in cerebral and cerebellar dendritic branching compared to mother-reared monkeys. The monkeys are thought to develop post-synaptic hypersensitivity, so that they have an over-response to a modest rise in CSF noradrenaline triggered by stress, leading to hyperaggressive reactions.

Behavioural abnormalities included an 'isolation syndrome' similar to that seen in human autism, schizophrenia, antisocial personality and explosive violence syndrome. Antipsychotic drugs and teaching foraging tasks reduce abnormal behaviours but do not improve social behaviours. In addition, these monkeys have specific cognitive deficits and show a despair-like response to later separation (Kraemer, 1992).

Care from 'therapist' peers has had the most impact on damaged monkeys, although it can be difficult to set up because of the aggression of the previously separated monkeys. Monkeys thus treated and rehabilitated are able to live alongside normally reared monkeys under non-stressful conditions, and to interact with them in an acceptable way. They continue to show cognitive abnormalities and despair responses to separation. If stressed, rehabilitated monkeys cannot find coping strategies and are liable to become aggressive.

These infant animals have been very severely deprived; it is rare to find a human infant who has had quite such an extreme experience. In studying the human infant we cannot be so cavalier in setting up experiments to isolate the baby or in removing bits of brain to study biogenic amines. We therefore have to be cautious in assuming too much about human development on the basis of animal experiments, although it is plausible to think that there may be parallels between this research and the effect of very severe deprivation on the immature human brain and mind.

We do not yet know the extent to which damage in the early years can be remedied in human children. It may be that very severe environmental failure at this early stage is irremediable, although presumably it is a matter of degree. We may have to accept that what the most damaged people need is a reliable and calm environment which will not stress them beyond what they can bear. Maybe as clinicians working with such people we can offer some help with drug treatment and psychotherapeutic intervention, but we should be limited and realistic in our therapeutic ambition.

The effect of experience on the mature brain

MAIN POINTS

- New learning can take place in adults.

- Animal research shows that brain changes accompany new learning.

- Psychosocial interventions must work by adding neural connections to existing ones.

We know from our own experience that new learning can take place in adults. Animal experiments have demonstrated both anatomical brain changes as a result of new learning and intracellular neurotransmitter change following new learning (Kandel *et al.*, 1995).

Again, research to date has only been possible in animals. In one series of experiments monkeys were trained to feed using only three fingers. After several weeks of this modified behaviour, the parts of the brain which represented the used fingers had enlarged and the parts representing the unused fingers had become smaller.

The complexity of the primate nervous system makes detailed study of specific change difficult, and so a simpler organism has been used to investigate change at a cellular level. The sea snail *Aplysia*, which has a very simple nervous system, has been extensively studied to explore the synaptic changes which accompany new learning. Studies of learning in *Aplysia* showed that new learning was accompanied by consistent changes in synaptic transmission and structural changes in the cells, and that the behavioural change and structural change persisted for up to several weeks.

Although the brain is at its most adaptive in early life, learning is an ability we do not lose. In an adult animal, new learning is accompanied by changes in effectiveness of neural connections. Thus when a person learns a new way of relating to others, or changes his self-image in relation to other people, there must be a corresponding change in neural connections within the brain. These changes may take place because of social experience or in the setting of a psychological treatment.

The nature of mental representations

MAIN POINTS

- Experience is laid down in the brain as neurally encoded mental representations.

- Not all experience is represented as verbally encoded memory.

- Verbal memory is not possible until the end of the second year of postnatal life when the prefrontal cortex is adequately mature.

- Experience in the first two years is important in the development of a well-functioning prefrontal cortex.

- Preverbal experience may be encoded as bodily memory, but this is speculative.

- Even verbal memory is not always historically accurate and is subject to potential distortion.

- Mental representation of self, the world and the relationships between oneself and others is the working model we bring to new situations.

- Mental representation is built up from our coding of experience in the mind and is not the same as historical memory.

- Experience is both external and internal, including thoughts, imaginings, memories and dreams.

continued ...

> • Mental representation is influenced by the person's interpretation of experience, and the laying down of mental representations will be affected by a child's developmental stage and by his understanding of external and internal events based on previous experience.

Mental representations are our working model of self in the world. They include codings for self, others, the relationship between these and a related emotional component. These are neurally represented.

Mental representations are built up from experience which includes:

• external experience in the world

• internal experience including thoughts, imagining, memories and dreams.

In the first two years, social interaction is essential for healthy mental development (Schore, 1994). The way in which the prefrontal cortex develops, and thus its efficient functioning, depend on the quality of experience the child has during that time, yet the brain is not yet capable of laying down memories which can be revived verbally. The child under two is capable of recognition, however, and of mentally organising experience on the basis of associations including affect, otherwise no social interaction would be possible.

Verbal memory depends on the effective functioning of the prefrontal cortex which is not biologically mature enough to verbally represent experience until the end of the second postnatal year. The prefrontal cortex organises verbal representation of experience and attaches words to memories.

Preverbal experience does have some representation in the brain, but it is relatively unorganised. It may be that such experience can have bodily expression as in psychosomatic symptoms, and that some apparently inexplicable states of arousal may be expressions of 'memory' of early distress. The despair response found in severely deprived monkeys is likely to be such a response to an experience which triggers a non-verbal 'memory' accompanied by a particular neurochemical state. We can see, however, that this is not what we usually mean by conventional memory, but is a behavioural re-enactment and biological response to a recognised but unnameable stimulus.

Accessible, verbally encoded memory begins at around two and a half to three years. Even then, however, we should not expect historical accuracy.

Actual experience whether internal or external is always *interpreted* by the individual and modified by two factors:

- the developmental level of the child

- the individual's previous experience which will colour the way in which he interprets and represents present experience.

Thus what gets represented in the mind is not always exactly what historically happened, but what the child or adult made of it. We may reasonably assume that mental representation bears some relation to actual experience, but as clinicians we must remember that memory is not a completely reliable instrument.

Because mental representations contribute to the organisation of present behaviour, we want to access mental representations in psychotherapy. *Reconstruction of actual events is relevant but less important,* and must always be somewhat conditional.

Mental representations and relating to the world

MAIN POINTS

- We use our mental representations as working models to guide our behaviour in new situations.

- We arrive in new situations with expectations based on our mental representations of situations which we identify as similar.

continued ...

- We may give unconscious signals to other people which indicate how we expect them to behave. This increases the likelihood of our getting the response we expect.

- We can modify existing working models to take account of new information. This is equivalent to new learning.

- Many people have difficulty in changing at least some of their working models, although rationally it would make sense to do so. Our motives for clinging to maladaptive behaviour are complex.

We use our mental representations as internal working models which provide a prototype to guide our behaviour when we encounter a new but similar situation. Previous experience leads to the development of expectations of ourselves and others in particular settings, and we tend not only to expect certain responses from other people but even to try to elicit them. (See also, The therapeutic relationship, p. 76.)

This is not to say that we cannot modify our previous behaviour and previous response in the light of new information. However, there appear to be times when we have difficulty in doing this and we cling, apparently irrationally, to our habitual ways of relating. To an extent, the ability to respond flexibly to new situations and to be able to think about change in oneself and others is a measure of mental health.

It was the observation of this apparent need to hold on to maladaptive behaviour which led Freud to postulate the existence of unconscious motives for some symptoms and behaviours.

References

Kandel ER, Schwartz JH and Jessell TM (1995) *Essentials of Neural Science and Behavior*. Appleton & Lange, Stamford, Connecticut. See especially Chapter 36, Cellular mechanisms of learning and memory, pp. 667–94.

Kraemer GW (1992) A psychobiological theory of attachment. *Behavioral and Brain Sciences.* **15**: 493–541.

Schore AN (1994) *Affect Regulation and the Origin of the Self: the neurobiology of emotional development.* Lawrence Erlbaum, Hillsdale, New Jersey.

Solms M (1997) Is the brain more real than the mind? *Psychoanalytic Psychotherapy.* **9**(2): 107–20.

Further reading

Greenfield S (ed) (1996) *The Human Mind Explained: the control centre of the living machine.* Cassell, London.

2

The psychodynamic in general psychiatry

Introduction • Meaning and disease in mental states • Causes and classification of mental disorder • Treatment of psychological problems: summary

Introduction

This chapter looks at some basic premises in our thinking in general psychiatry and suggests where a dynamic approach might integrate into the practice of psychiatry. It does not address issues related to the management of severe mental illness, in particular where the patient is a danger to himself or other people. Nor does it begin to look at a multitude of important issues in general psychiatry, such as the role of the multidisciplinary team, community management or social interventions.

Meaning and disease in mental states

MAIN POINTS

- We use different models of the mind when we conceptualise mental disorder. These include the disease model and the meaning model.

- The disease model focuses on anatomical and physiological malfunctioning in the person.

- The meaning model assumes that mental states have psychological meaning for the individual even when he is suffering some form of mental disorder.

- These two models are not mutually exclusive and the medical model should be one which integrates them.

- The treatment of the patient may address the symptoms, both in terms of the physical malfunctioning and in terms of the meaning of the symptoms for the patient.

Diagnosis and diagnostic categories: There are advantages and disadvantages to using diagnostic categories and there are different ways of classifying mental disorder.

The disease model: The disease model classifies disorder on the basis of symptom clusters which assume underlying anatomical and physiological change, and imply that there is a unitary disease process corresponding to the symptoms. This is the neuropathology of a disorder. Using classification like this allows relatively easy communication between professionals, standardisation of research, and prediction about the course of a particular disease. The weakness of the model lies in its power to explain individual human behaviour.

The meaning model: The meaning model gives less significance to diagnostic categories. Instead, it emphasises the importance of the psychological organisation deriving from the person's experience and internal (mental) model of the world, and assumes that mental states have personal meaning. This meaning is described in the psychopathology of a problem. The model uses a descriptive approach, recognising individual differences. The strength of this model is its explanatory power in understanding human behaviour. Its weakness is that the limited use of diagnostic groups reduces the ease with which research can be done and with which firm predictions can be made.

In everyday life, we tend to assume that emotional states or behaviours have meaning: '*I am anxious about my exam*'. This makes good sense to us. At times we may think that there is something abnormal about an emotion, that it is either excessive or is not appropriate to the problem.

'*I feel sick with anxiety all the time, doctor. I can hardly go out of the house because of it. I lost my job because I missed so many days when I couldn't manage to leave the house. I need something for it.*'

This person is not attributing any meaningful stimulus to his anxiety. He feels he is suffering an abnormal state which he connects to some physiological malfunctioning. And in a way he is right: abnormal states of arousal do have a physical component, although we may also think it likely that even in this case there must be some meaningful external or internal event which is acting as a trigger to the anxiety.

   Is it possible to both regard the response as inappropriate and also to attribute personal meaning to a state of anxiety?

While shopping with her mother three-year-old Bella runs on to the road and is hit by a car. She suffers a fractured femur, but eventually makes a full recovery. Her mother, however, remains intensely anxious about her safety and will not allow her to go to nursery school for fear of another accident.

The mother's anxiety is excessive but understandable. We may think that perhaps she feels guilt about what happened and that she also sees the world as a dangerous and threatening place.

From the day she became pregnant Mrs Smith was afraid that something would happen to her baby. She had a straightforward pregnancy and uncomplicated delivery, but remained anxious about her child's health and made frequent visits to the GP with him. She would not allow him to attend nursery in case he caught an infection.

Mrs Smith's anxiety is excessive and more difficult to understand. If we want to make sense of it we must look for meanings which are not reasonable and not entirely conscious. She also sees the world as threatening and dangerous to her child, but we cannot immediately see why this should be.

When we treat a patient who is suffering painful emotional symptoms, we need to consider at which level we are going to intervene, and whether this person will best be served by our trying to remove symptoms chemically or by a psychological intervention which will include establishing the meaning of the symptoms for the patient. Some patients and some problems do best with some combination of the two. (See also, A dynamic formulation of psychiatric diagnoses, p. 84.)

Causes and classification of mental disorder

MAIN POINTS

- In clinical practice the causes of mental disorder can be usefully subdivided into predisposing, precipitating and maintaining factors.

- The absence of a reliable test for most mental disorders means that classification depends on clinical judgement of observed and reported symptoms.

- It is likely that within larger categories there are disorders which have clinical similarity but may have different causes and different underlying pathology.

- Many people who seek psychological help are not suffering from one clear problem which falls easily into one diagnostic category.

- The multifactorial causes of most mental illnesses suggest that different approaches to treatment may be useful, including pharmacological, psychological and social.

When we consider causes of mental disorder in clinical situations it is useful to think of:

- predisposing factors
- precipitating factors
- maintaining factors.

Predisposing factors

- Genetic loading.
- Early environmental impact on the immature organism leading to constitutional vulnerability, either biological and/or psychological.

Precipitating factors

- Current environmental stressors.
- Biological factors, e.g. infection, degeneration etc, or change in brain function of unknown cause.

Maintaining factors

- Family or social factors.
- Habitual patterns of relating: familiar or learned behaviours.
- Secondary gain, conscious or unconscious.
- Physiological change in the brain.

All these factors, the predisposing, precipitating and maintaining, contribute to the clinical presentation which the patient brings to the doctor. The patient complains of psychological and sometimes physical symptoms, for which we can assume there will be an underlying pathological change. This pathology is likely to be both neuronal and psychological.

The pathology of much mental disturbance is only partly understood. For example, we may assume that low mood is accompanied by neurochemical change in the central nervous system (CNS). But as yet we do not have the means of distinguishing any difference between the change which accompanies normal sadness and the low mood which accompanies severe depressive disorder. We simply do not know if these are quite different processes or if the disorder is an extreme of the normal process.

To illustrate the various contributions of different causative factors to mental illness, and the pathology which results, let us take the example of depression.

Scenario 1

Let us postulate that John is born with a genetic coding which makes him vulnerable to mood change. When the usual monoamine changes of stress occur, most people have some regulatory process which allows the normal state to return within a few days. With genetically vulnerable individuals like John there is a danger that following stress or perhaps as a result of some as yet unidentified spontaneous process in the brain, a change of the level of CNS monoamines will not spontaneously return to normal and the individual will develop a depressive illness.

The cause of John's depression is largely genetic, though current life stressors may have played an aetiological part in his current episode of illness.

The *psychological symptoms* are low mood, self-blaming thoughts, etc. The *somatic symptoms* are sleep disturbance, appetite disturbance, lack of energy, etc. The *neuropathology*, so far as we understand it, is fall in noradrenaline in his CNS and as yet unidentified synaptic changes. To get an understanding of the *psychopathology* (mental representations) we need more information about John's personality, his behaviour and thoughts and his present and past life experience.

Scenario 2

James is born with a normal genetic coding for mood regulation. He is not genetically vulnerable to low mood. He was the child of a 17-year-old single mother. She found him a more taxing infant than she expected and her new boyfriend was frankly antagonistic. When he was 14 months old he was suspected of having suffered non-accidental injury and was below the third centile for his weight. After a year's fostering he was returned to his mother, now married to her boyfriend. At six years he and his younger sisters were removed from the parents and the stepfather served a five-year custodial sentence for physical cruelty to the children. By this time James was behaviourally disturbed and he spent the remainder of his childhood in fostering placements which broke down, and in children's homes. From late teens he suffered episodes of depression.

James did not start out with genetic vulnerability, but he acquired vulnerability. We may speculate that this is constitutional, and has resulted from the impact of the non-nurturing and frightening early environment on his immature neural circuitry. He did not suffer what would be called 'brain damage' in the conventional sense, but we may wonder if his brain development was nonetheless impaired. His ability to deal with the ordinary stresses of life is limited. His ability to form stable relationships is limited. He gets depressed when he feels helpless, which is often. It is likely that this is a different process from the scenario of genetic inheritance.

The cause of James's depression is early developmental damage and current life stresses. The *psychological symptoms* are depressed mood, self-blaming thoughts, etc. The *somatic symptoms* are lack of energy, poor concentration, anxiety, etc. The *neuropathology* can only be speculated, but is possibly poor CNS regulation of monoamines. The *psychopathology* will be complex, but is likely to include expectations of abuse and fractured relationships, and a sense of himself as unlovable and perhaps dangerous.

Scenario 3

Jack does not have the strong genetic loading for vulnerability to mood change which John has. He is the second of two children and had what he describes as a normal childhood, brought up by both parents in fairly comfortable circumstances. He was close to his mother, who had always been rather shy and did not have many friends. Jack trained as a teacher and lived at home with his parents until he married at the age of 24 years. The marriage was not a success and two years later he returned to live with his parents. He soon became depressed and sought help from his family doctor. He made a moderate response to antidepressants but returned six months later with a relapse of his symptoms.

Jack is the kind of patient whom we meet often in the GP surgery or a psychiatry outpatient clinic. The causes of Jack's depression are multiple, and may include genetic factors, factors deriving from the early environment and current stresses, including family issues. A maintaining factor may be a degree of unconscious secondary gain from his being depressed. The *psychological symptoms* are low mood, thoughts of helplessness, etc. The *somatic symptoms* are poor sleep, lack of energy, etc. The *neuropathology* is presumably some change in neurotransmitters, but possibly not the same changes which affect either John or James. The *psychopathology* is speculative without knowing Jack better, but hypothetically may include a sense of helplessness and anger over an inability to resolve the conflict over his wish to be close to his parents and protective of his mother, and his wish for independence.

These scenarios raise several issues:

- The definition of depression: symptom, symptom cluster and diagnosis.

- The absence of a test for 'depression' leaves us dependent on clinical presentation and symptom cluster, observable and reported. Thus it is possible that we subsume conditions which have different causes and different pathology under the diagnostic classification of 'depression'.

- It seems likely that depressed mood is accompanied by biological change, but can we assume a final common biological pathway for all causes of depressed mood?

Clinical experience suggests that symptoms can be addressed on several different fronts:

- the chemical or pharmacological: modifying neurotransmitter action within the brain

- the cognitive: modifying conscious or almost conscious thoughts which maintain low mood

- the level of mental representation: clarifying the representations of self and others which maintain depression, i.e. the secondary gain which may not be fully conscious

- the level of family or social interaction, which may be maintaining symptoms

- the societal: issues related to things like housing, employment, crime, which have a relevant impact on the person.

For any patient, even John with his strong genetic loading, all five of these may contribute to the modification of current symptoms and the prevention of future episodes.

There are very few mental disorders for which there is a reliable test, and most disturbances could be considered in the way outlined above, postulating a 'core' of individuals who have a strong genetic loading and a larger group with similar symptoms for whom genetic predisposition plays a smaller part. In virtually all cases, however, we may assume that several factors contribute to the onset of the illness. Causes are multiple, and the situation is further complicated by the fact that, once established, disorders will have maintaining factors both within the individual and in his environment.

In treating patients, we need to consider at which level we are going to intervene, and whether the patient will best be served by our trying to remove symptoms chemically or by a psychological intervention which will include establishing the meaning of the symptoms for the patient. Some patients and some problems do best with some combination of the two. (See also, A dynamic formulation of psychiatric diagnoses, p. 84.)

Treatment of psychological problems: summary

MAIN POINTS

- Most mental disturbance is caused by several factors, past and current.

- The impact on the person is often partly physiological and partly psychological. This is reflected in the symptoms.

- Mental disturbance can be treated at a pharmacological level, at a personal psychological level and at a family or social level. Sometimes treatment includes intervention at all three levels.

We have seen that most emotional problems and mental disturbances have multiple determinants, including innate (genetic) predisposition and the earlier experience that leads to mental representations of the world and the relationships the person therefore expects. In addition, more often than not we find that an episode of mental disturbance is triggered by an external or internal event which has meaning for the person. The meaning may be in the present or may remind the person of some associated memory or previous experience.

States of mind have organisation at different levels, which are anatomical, neurochemical and psychological. In each clinical situation we have to decide whether a patient will be best helped by physical (drugs) or psychological intervention or a combination of the two.

Further reading

Bolton D and Hill J (1996) *Mind, Meaning and Mental Disorder: the nature of causal explanation in psychology and psychiatry.* Oxford University Press, Oxford.

3

What is psychotherapy?

Definition of psychotherapy • Characteristics of all psychotherapies • Classification of the psychotherapies • Problem-solving or not? • Behavioural psychotherapy • Cognitive psychotherapy • Psychodynamic psychotherapy (also called psychoanalytic psychotherapy) • Interpersonal therapy • Counselling • Systemic therapy (family therapy) • What is the difference between cognitive psychotherapy and psychodynamic psychotherapy? • What is the difference between counselling and psychodynamic psychotherapy?

MAIN POINTS

- Psychotherapy is a blanket term for those treatments which offer psychological rather than physical or social intervention.

- The psychotherapies share some common characteristics.

- Those usually available on the NHS include behavioural, cognitive, psychodynamic and interpersonal therapies, counselling and systemic or family therapies.

- Some focus on specific problems and others look more broadly at patterns of behaviour, thoughts and feelings.

continued ...

- Behaviour therapy aims to reduce symptoms by changing specific behaviours.

- Cognitive therapy aims to reduce symptoms by changing thoughts which maintain specific symptoms.

- Psychodynamic therapy aims to change habitual patterns of thinking, feeling and behaviour which may include specific symptoms.

- Interpersonal therapy aims to help the patient identify and find solutions to current life problems and has been mainly used for depression.

- Counselling aims to offer a supportive, non-directive relationship in which the patient can work out solutions to personal difficulties.

- Family therapy aims to see if and how the problem of the identified patient is maintained by the needs of the family.

Definition of psychotherapy

Psychotherapy is the treatment of emotional, behavioural or personality problems by psychological means.

Although different techniques may be used to treat the problems, the object in any psychotherapeutic treatment is to bring some change in feelings, thoughts, attitudes or behaviours which have been troublesome to the patient. The treatment aims to relieve symptoms and to help the person think for himself and become more satisfied with his life.

This chapter gives an overview of psychotherapies currently practised in the NHS and indicates how psychodynamic psychotherapy relates to these.

Characteristics of all psychotherapies

- An intense, emotionally charged, *confiding relationship* with a helping person.

- A rationale which contains an *explanation* of the patient's distress and of the methods for its release.

- The provision of *new information* about the nature and origins of the patient's problems and of ways of dealing with them.

- *Hope* in the patient that he can expect help from the therapy.

- An opportunity for experiences of success during the course of therapy and a consequent enhancement of the *sense of mastery*.

- The facilitation of *emotional arousal* in the patient.

Jerome Frank (1971)

Classification of the psychotherapies

This section outlines the kinds of psychotherapy generally available in the National Health Service. There are other psychological interventions, some reputable and some of dubious provenance, which are less well known or less widely available, but these will not be discussed here.

It is important to remember that a therapist may be trained to practice more than one kind of psychotherapy, and that an experienced practitioner will often use more than one technique with one patient or one problem. The psychotherapies commonly available in the NHS include:

- behavioural psychotherapy

- cognitive psychotherapy

- psychodynamic (psychoanalytic) psychotherapy

- interpersonal therapy

- counselling
- systemic therapy (family therapy).

Problem-solving or not?

Psychotherapies are sometimes classified on the basis of the balance between actively addressing specific problems and non-judgemental, non-directive listening. Cognitive, behavioural and interpersonal therapies are very clearly problem-focused, and the therapist will stick to his remit to address a particular problem. These therapies are overtly directive in that, having agreed a goal, the therapist will maintain a focus and bring the patient back to the focus when necessary.

Psychodynamic therapies are not directly problem-solving, but are active treatments. Short-term psychodynamic therapy also seeks a specific focus and concentrates on this in much the same way as interpersonal therapy. Longer-term psychodynamic therapy does not seek a single and specific focus, but is active in the sense that the therapist analyses the material which the patient brings to the session and expects the patient to be active in doing the same.

It is difficult to be specific about counselling, because the term does not cover a single technique. Counselling may be non-directive and predominantly the provision of a supportive listening relationship in which the client explores personal difficulties. It may also be problem-focused, however, incorporating techniques from both interpersonal therapy and psychodynamic therapy.

Behavioural psychotherapy

Behaviour therapy is based on learning theory. The focus of treatment is on changing behaviour, rather than feelings and thoughts (Stern and Drummond, 1991). As with physical treatments the primary aim is symptom relief rather than an attempt to understand the mental representations which are sustaining the symptoms. The behaviour therapist is not concerned with the reasons behind the symptoms, whether these be irrational thoughts or unconscious fears.

The theoretical view is that neurotic symptoms are examples of maladaptive behaviour and result from faulty learning. The goal of treatment is to unlearn specific patterns of behaviour and, through new learning, to replace them with more adaptive patterns. The main obstacle to changing maladaptive behaviour is that the person feels intensely anxious when he attempts change.

Asking for behaviour change of a person who has a particular fear, for example a phobic fear of flying, increases anxiety painfully. The art of behavioural intervention is to modify behaviour gradually and at a rate which allows anxiety to remain at tolerable levels. Therapy makes active use of the notion of reward or positive experience in reinforcing behaviours.

Behavioural treatment is the most effective treatment for:

- obsessive compulsive disorder (OCD)
- specific phobias
- some sexual disorders.

Patients with OCD and specific phobias should always be referred for behaviour therapy in the first instance.

Cognitive psychotherapy

Cognitive therapy is concerned with the way in which maladaptive behaviour or feelings may be reinforced by thoughts (Beck, 1995). A person who is suffering from, say, depression, may interpret/misinterpret many things in his environment in such a negative way that his self-esteem sinks steadily lower. The cognitive therapist will challenge this thinking and ask the patient to identify the thoughts which are maintaining the depressed mood and to re-evaluate the assumptions he is making.

The cognitive approach is particularly useful for patients who have a specific symptom, such as depressed mood, which can be the focus of a relatively short-term therapy. Cognitive therapy may be useful in the treatment of:

- depression

- anxiety states

- long-standing delusions and hallucinations in schizophrenia.

None of these diagnoses is an absolute indication for cognitive therapy and the decision about whether the person will benefit from cognitive treatment depends on other factors, such as other symptoms, motivation and the wishes of the patient. The treatment of people with long-standing delusions or hallucinations is fairly new and some, though not all, patients with these symptoms benefit from this approach.

Patients who have a fairly unambiguous interest in getting better and who are highly cooperative are more likely to do well in cognitive therapy than those who have mixed feelings or motives.

Psychodynamic psychotherapy (also called psychoanalytic psychotherapy)

Psychodynamic psychotherapy is concerned with the way in which a person's mental representation of self and the world may lead to inappropriate behaviour in present personal and working relationships. This approach seeks a personal meaning for the patient's symptoms in terms of his or her past and present life. It emphasises the importance of mental representations of earlier life experiences in the present, the conscious and unconscious expectations which these 'working models' bring to relationships, and the way in which the person may unconsciously invite others to play a role in his expected scenario.

Psychodynamic psychotherapy aims to help the patient by increasing understanding of his thoughts, feelings and behaviour. It is sometimes called 'exploratory' or 'insight directed' therapy. It is helpful for patients with a wide range of emotional disorders.

Patients usually seek dynamic psychotherapy or are referred for therapy if they recognise that they have interpersonal problems as well as symptoms, and if they can see that this pervades their lives and are prepared to work to change themselves. Diagnostic conditions in which a person may seek dynamic therapy include:

- depression

- anxiety disorder

- personality disorder

- eating disorder.

The list of diagnoses may be somewhat misleading. As with cognitive therapy, not all people with these diagnoses will find this approach useful. In reality, few patients come for therapy with a single diagnosis and most have long-standing personality problems in addition to their primary diagnosis.

Behavioural, cognitive and psychodynamic therapies can all be stressful treatments and the patient needs to be able to tolerate and work with a certain amount of anxiety. The training and experience of the therapist are important in helping him assess how much anxiety the patient can cope with at any time, and in ensuring that this remains at a level where the patient can work effectively.

Interpersonal therapy

Interpersonal psychotherapy helps a person to clarify current problems and find the best way of dealing with them (Weissman and Markowitz, 1994). It has mainly been used for depression. It is a brief therapy (usually no more than 15 sessions). The therapist focuses on the patient's present situation and present relationship to identify the triggers to the depressive episode and the factors which may be maintaining the symptoms.

Interpersonal therapy shares some aspects of dynamic psychotherapy in that the therapist helps the patient see how his present way of relating to other people and expectations of relationships may have contributed to his depression. The therapy does not, however, explore the past. The therapist is active both in identifying problem areas and working with the patient in finding alternative strategies to deal with depression in the future.

Counselling

Counselling is used here to describe a non-directive approach, in which the therapist offers support and non-judgemental listening, to facilitate the patient finding solutions to personal difficulties. The therapist will recognise the importance of previous life experience in how the patient is dealing with his problems, and may use this to help the patient make sense of how he is dealing with current issues.

In general, this approach is less stressful than other kinds of therapy. It is not intended to make the patient confront his anxieties so much as to strengthen existing coping strategies and find new ones. The therapist may give sympathy and encouragement.

In the NHS, counselling is commonly used for three kinds of patient:

- those who consult their GP with mild to moderate psychological problems such as symptoms of depression or anxiety
- those who usually cope adequately but have had a life crisis which is not resolving in the usual way, e.g. a prolonged bereavement reaction
- hospital patients who have particular illnesses, e.g. those suffering from cancer or AIDS.

Counselling is a poorly defined term, and is often loosely used to mean any non-directive or non-challenging approach. Although such research as there is shows non-directive counselling to be no better than 'treatment as usual', it is popular with patients, and the research findings reflect the difficulty in defining appropriate outcome measures in psychotherapy research (see below).

Systemic therapy (family therapy)

Systemic therapy has come to be more or less synonymous with family therapy. It is based on the assumption that a symptom or interpersonal problem can and sometimes should be addressed within the social context in which it arises. The therapy aims to identify the function of the presenting symptom or problem in maintaining the family system, and to help the family identify alternative and more adaptive ways in which family needs can be satisfied.

Family therapy is an appropriate treatment:

- for childhood problems where one or more children in a family are showing behavioural or emotional difficulties within their family or where problems at school appear to be related to family difficulties

- during adolescence and early adulthood where young people with psychiatric, psychological or emotional difficulties are still strongly bound up with their families or origin

- at other stages in the family life cycle:

  - when family members are showing signs of problems in dealing with their relationships with each other

  - when a family has persistent difficulty negotiating a life problem, such as sickness, bereavement or divorce

  - where an individual appears to have a psychiatric, psychological or emotional problem which affects and is affected by other members of his family.

What is the difference between cognitive psychotherapy and psychodynamic psychotherapy?

MAIN POINTS

- Cognitive therapy works on a single symptom, on conscious thoughts, and seeks a rational alternative to irrational thinking.

- Psychodynamic therapy works on patterns of thoughts, feelings and behaviours, and suggests that apparently irrational behaviour may have a 'rational' unconscious motive. The therapy therefore attempts to access unconscious as well as conscious thoughts and feelings.

- Cognitive therapy does not use the therapeutic relationship as an active part of the treatment. Psychodynamic therapy uses analysis of the therapeutic relationship to explore the patient's conscious and unconscious expectations and model of the world.

- Both challenge maladaptive patterns of thinking and irrational assumptions.

- The cognitive therapist usually focuses on a single symptom, such as depressed mood, while the dynamic therapist will address the wider question of patterns of maladaptive behaviour in several areas of the patient's life.

- The cognitive therapist is interested in conscious or accessible thoughts, which maintain symptoms. The dynamic therapist may also seek to find the unconscious thoughts and feelings which may contain motives which support maladaptive behaviour.

- The dynamic therapist is interested in why a patient may cling to his symptoms for reasons which he does not understand. It is this apparently irrational behaviour which leads the dynamic therapist to suggest that when there is no rational and conscious reason maintaining the symptoms there may be unconscious thoughts or feelings underlying the problem.

- The cognitive therapist maintains a friendly, non-judgemental relationship with the patient, but does not use the therapeutic relationship as an active part of the treatment. The dynamic psychotherapist uses the analysis of the therapeutic relationship as a way to access and understand non-conscious as well as conscious parts of the patient's expectations and model of the world.

What is the difference between counselling and psychodynamic psychotherapy?

MAIN POINTS

- Counselling and dynamic psychotherapy are related but not identical skills, and one person may be qualified to practise both.

- Counselling offers non-judgemental support and encourages the person to clarify and prioritise current problems, and to find solutions. Negative feelings in the therapeutic relationship are not usually explored.

- Psychodynamic therapy is supportive but does not directly help to solve problems. It seeks to understand the person's state of mind, how he contributes to his own difficulties, actively uses the therapeutic relationship to understand unconscious thoughts and feelings, and accepts that there will be negative feelings to be understood in the relationship.

In medical practice, counselling is welcomed by patients who generally believe that talking about one's problems is useful. Counselling gets a mixed response from doctors, some of whom who see it as non-scientific and, because its effect is difficult to quantify empirically, of dubious worth.

There is often confusion between counselling and psychotherapy because the terms are sometimes used interchangeably. We find people who have had a long and rigorous training in dynamic psychotherapy employed as 'counsellors' in general practice and, on the other hand, people who have done a few weeks' course in so-called counselling or psychotherapy setting up practice as 'psychotherapists'.

The issue of training and who is qualified to practise in which way is discussed on p. 123. A person may be trained to do both counselling and dynamic psychotherapy and a skilled practitioner will make a judgement about when to take one or other approach with a patient. In practice, although there is a model of counselling which is truly non-directive, most skilled counsellors use a combination of non-judgemental listening and problem-solving.

In this author's view, good counselling includes:

- clarifying present problems and helping quantify and prioritise them

- encouraging the person to identify the source of the present difficulties so as to understand how the situation arose

- if necessary, helping the patient seek for explanations in the past which may contribute to present problems

- helping the person identify possible solutions to the problems

- helping the person identify sources of support and help in his life

- maintaining a mildly friendly and positive relationship, with encouragement and advice, so that the person feels supported and more able to solve his present difficulties.

In general, in counselling the therapist will not explore past experience in depth, nor use the analysis of the therapeutic relationship to understand the patient's unconscious mental representations. The development of negative feelings which are then to be understood and explored (worked through) is not part of a counselling therapy. Most counselling is fairly short term and non-intensive, and takes place once a week or less for a number of weeks or months.

The psychodynamic therapist is also supportive and friendly, but will not usually help directly with solving specific problems, although she may work on why the patient puts obstacles in the way of finding available solutions. The therapist seeks to recognise and understand the patient's states of mind, rather than offering solutions to problems. The therapist also analyses the patient's behaviour, thoughts and feelings, i.e. examines their meaning, in terms of the patient's needs and wishes, conscious and unconscious.

In a psychodynamic therapy:

- The therapist is supportive of the patient, but will be cautious about being drawn into a relationship where she offers to solve the patient's problems. The implicit refusal to behave as expected or to offer solutions when they are asked for often allows identification of certain expectations in the patient.

- The therapist pays particular attention to recognising and acknowledging the patient's state of mind, both positive and negative. This recognition and sense of being understood should not be underrated. It is often experienced by the patient as calming and therapeutic.

- Along with less emphasis on direct problem-solving, there is more emphasis on why the problems have arisen, what the patient himself has contributed to this, and in analysing any obstacles that he creates to finding feasible solutions. Possible unconscious as well as conscious motives are explored.

- The therapist will actively use the therapeutic relationship to explore the patient's negative as well as positive feelings in the therapy, and his irrational as well as rational feelings and fantasies about himself and other people, including the therapist.

Psychodynamic psychotherapy is useful for people with longer-standing problems who have suffered from interpersonal difficulties for a long period, usually many years, and who appear to have the ability to 'shoot themselves in the foot', i.e. to sabotage their own lives, even without outside help. Psychodynamic psychotherapy aims to give the patient enough understanding about himself to know what he has contributed to having the problems, to find possible alternatives and to give him a choice of continuing to use the same ways of dealing with relationships and life, or of using new ways which may serve him better.

There is no absolute line between counselling and dynamic therapy. In bereavement counselling, for example, it will be essential to explore the relationship with the lost person and it may be important to identify possible unconscious feelings, such as anger to this person which may be contributing to the delay in resolution of mourning. This counselling, however, would be focused on that particular relationship and would probably not explore either previous relationships in childhood or the feelings which the patient may have for the counsellor.

References

Beck JS (1995) *Cognitive Therapy: basics and beyond.* Guilford Press, Hove.

Frank J (1971) Therapeutic factors in psychotherapy. *American Journal of Psychotherapy.* **25**: 350–61.

Stern R and Drummond L (1991) *The Practice of Behavioural and Cognitive Psychotherapy.* Cambridge University Press, Cambridge.

Weissman MM and Markowitz J (1994) Interpersonal psychotherapy: current status. *Archives of General Psychiatry.* **51**: 599–606.

Further reading

Brown D and Pedder J (1979) *Introduction to Psychotherapy.* Tavistock Publications, London.

Skinner R and Cleese J (1983) *Families and How to Survive Them.* Methuen, London.

4

Theory of psychodynamic psychotherapy

Introduction • The contribution of Sigmund Freud (1856–1939) • Freud's topographical theory and the unconscious mind • The concept of conflict • Freud's structural theory: the place of innate instincts • Eric Berne and transactional analysis (a modification of the structural theory) • Freud's developmental theory: early determinants of personality and behaviour • The Oedipus complex • The present status of Freud's ideas • The contribution of Melanie Klein • Attachment theory and attachment behaviour • Psychological defence mechanisms • The therapeutic relationship: working alliance, transference and countertransference • Other psychoanalytic terms used in psychodynamic psychotherapy • A dynamic formulation of psychiatric diagnoses

Introduction

This is a highly selected and brief outline of some of the most important theoretical ideas in psychoanalytic psychotherapy. Many of these ideas originated with Sigmund Freud, who has been a major figure in 20th century thought, not only in psychiatry but in literature, history and anthropology. Some of Freud's ideas which are well known but not now entirely accepted are described, and later developments are mentioned alongside them.

The contribution of Sigmund Freud (1856–1939)

MAIN POINTS

- As a neurologist, Freud was aware that some physical symptoms did not relate to the neuroanatomical structures serving the afflicted area.

- He proposed that psychological organisation might sometimes take precedence over anatomical in symptom development.

- Freud outlined three main theories to account for mental process: the topographical, the structural and the developmental.

- Although psychoanalysis and psychodynamic psychotherapy have changed a lot since Freud's time, many of his ideas have been the starting point for further theoretical and clinical developments.

Freud trained as a physiologist and a physician, and was accustomed to using the clinical anatomical method to understand how his patients' symptoms related to the underlying pathological process. Using this method, a patient's symptoms were carefully recorded, and when he died the post-mortem would reveal the anatomical changes associated with the symptoms he had had in life. Gradually a picture was built up of the anatomical changes underlying particular diseases.

Freud became aware that this method did not always work when the patient was suffering from a nervous disease. This was particularly striking when the patient had a physical symptom which did not relate to the known anatomical structures serving the area. For example, a patient might have a paralysis of a limb which did not correspond to the known distribution of the nerves to that limb. Freud realised that the illness in this case was related not to an anatomical process but to a psychological one, and proposed that the functions of the mind are not always organised anatomically, but that they have a psychological organisation which is somewhat independent of a primary anatomical organisation.

Although Freud was not the first person to suggest that the mind is a dynamic entity, his outline of psychoanalysis as a theory and method of treatment has brought a systematic approach to psychodynamic therapy.

Psychoanalysis and psychodynamic psychotherapy have changed since Freud's time. Some of his concepts, however, have remained important in theory and practice, and even those that have been discarded as not clinically useful or accurate have often been a starting point for later clinicians and researchers to develop their ideas.

Three important ideas which have been influential in psychoanalysis and psychotherapy derive from Freud's three main theories:

1 That our behaviour is influenced by *unconscious* thoughts and feelings, and that symptoms may arise because of *conflict* between conscious thoughts and wishes and unconscious thoughts and wishes. This was part of Freud's topographical theory.

2 That we are born with *innate instincts* which affect our behaviour. This was part of Freud's structural theory.

3 That *early development* has an important influence on adult behaviour. This was part of Freud's developmental theory.

Freud's topographical theory and the unconscious mind

MAIN POINTS

- Freud was not the first person to suggest that there is an unconscious part of the human mind.

- Neuropsychological research in the late 20th century has confirmed that much mental process is outside conscious awareness.

continued ...

- Freud postulated that there are unconscious thoughts and feelings in the mind which may influence behaviour.

- A thought may be unconscious because it is consciously suppressed or it may be unconscious because it is unconsciously repressed.

Freud was not the first person to suggest the existence of an unconscious part of the mind. The psychologist Herbart and the philosopher Schopenhauer in the 19th century both anticipated Freud's ideas. In the later 20th century, neuropsychology has confirmed via subliminal perception and preconscious processing that much mental life takes place outside of awareness (Dixon and Henley, 1991).

Freud began with the rational premise that our feelings, behaviours, thoughts and symptoms are not random or arbitrary. There is some reason or meaning behind their happening. This assumption is called psychic determinism. If we believe that thoughts, feelings and behaviours are not random, but have some reason to be there, then we look for a cause which will explain them, or give meaning to them.

To give meaning to mental events (feelings, symptoms, behaviours) Freud postulated the existence of thoughts in the patient's mind which are unconscious but which can affect his conscious mind and behaviour. It may be preferable to think in terms of different levels of consciousness and use the word unconscious as an adjective rather than a noun. We can identify three kinds of unconscious thoughts:

1 Something may be unconscious because I happen not to be thinking of it at this moment, such as what I had for lunch last Sunday.

2 It may be unconscious because it is a painful memory which I consciously choose to suppress rather than remember, like the exam viva I made such a mess of. Freud used the word 'preconscious' to describe these levels of unconscious thought which are available to the conscious mind if we choose to look at them.

3 It may be unconscious because I have unconsciously repressed it and it therefore cannot be recalled at will. Freud suggested that an idea or a memory may be so painful to us, or may conflict with our view of ourselves in such a way that it would cause acute anxiety or guilt if it were acknowledged. From his experience as a doctor, Freud observed that repressed feelings could cause physical as well as psychological symptoms.

For example, a young man, Dave, suffers severe headaches after the sudden death of his much loved mother. After six months with no improvement, his general practitioner suggests they spend time thinking about his relationship with his mother and arranges four half-hour appointments with her patient. In the third session the GP suggests that Dave is angry with his mother for leaving him. The young man thinks about this and reluctantly agrees that this is possibly so. To his surprise his headaches disappear during the following few days.

Dave felt both love for his mother and anger with her because she had left him when he still felt he needed her. The feelings of anger conflicted with his view of how he ought to feel about his mother, and he repressed these unacceptable feelings. He suffered inexplicable tension, however, with painful headaches which only got better when his unacceptable conflictual feelings could be acknowledged.

The concept of conflict

MAIN POINTS

- The experience of having conflicting wishes is familiar to everyone.

- Conflict may be conscious or unconscious.

- According to Freud, unconscious conflict may lead to the development of symptoms.

We are all familiar with the experience of conscious conflict.

Mrs A wants to have her elderly mother to live with her rather than for her to go into a home for the elderly, but she knows that her mother hates noise and will make her young children's lives a misery. Mrs A wants to be a caring daughter and a caring mother and she cannot be both. She is in conflict.

Sometimes, as in the case of Dave, conflict is not conscious.

Mrs B wants to have her elderly mother to live with her. She has no children at home, but she has recently begun to have severe backaches which have led to her postponing her mother's move into her home.

Mrs B may be suffering from a physical back problem, but is it also possible that she could also be in conflict, this time unconscious conflict?

Freud's structural theory: the place of innate instincts

MAIN POINTS

- Freud suggested that the mind could be conceptualised as having three parts: the ego, the superego and the id.

- The ego is the rational part of the mind which accepts external reality and negotiates between the wishes and needs of the person and the demands of the outside world. The ego is mainly conscious.

- The superego is what we think of as conscience. It is part conscious and part unconscious. It may be helpful or punitive.

- The id is the part of the mind which contains the instincts of sexuality and aggression. It is mainly unconscious.

In 1923, Freud introduced his structural theory of the mind. He described the mind as having three parts, the ego, the superego and the id.

Roughly speaking:

- **Id** corresponds to the basic instincts of sex and aggression, and is largely unconscious.

- **Ego** corresponds to the rational, thinking part of the mind which recognises other people's needs as well as one's own and is largely conscious.

- **Superego** corresponds to what we would know as conscience and is built from identifications with important authority figures such as parents and teachers. Superego is part conscious and part unconscious.

According to this way of conceptualising the mind, the baby is born with strong instincts towards satisfaction (id instincts) and with no awareness of the needs of other people. Gradually, as he becomes more biologically mature, he begins to realise that there is a world out there and that his needs must be negotiated with those of other people. This is the beginning of what Freud called 'ego function'.

Also during the early years, the baby both realises and imagines that other people can be aggressive just like he can, and begins to fear that he could be hurt or punished if he offends someone. This is the beginning of the development of superego or conscience. This is a simplistic description of a complex idea developed by Freud as a way to understand how the mind works.

The term 'ego function' is sometimes used to refer to a person's capacity for rational thinking, and the term 'superego' is used in a psychoanalytic setting to denote the capacity for self-criticism. The term 'id' is less used now in either psychoanalysis or in psycho-therapy, and the notion of innate instincts seeking release has been modified to include ideas about how such feelings may develop in the context of relationships.

Eric Berne and transactional analysis (a modification of the structural theory)

> ## MAIN POINTS
>
> - Eric Berne used Freud's ideas of the ego, superego and id to develop an easily accessible formulation of how the mind works.
>
> - He proposed three parts to the mind which he called Adult, Parent and Child.
>
> - He incorporated the notion of mental representations so that each of these parts had an associated expected relationship or transaction.
>
> - His ideas have been widely used in the practice of transactional analysis.

A more easily accessible if somewhat bowdlerised version of Freud's structural model of the mind has been described by Eric Berne. His popular books (for example, *Games People Play* (1966)) are highly effective in showing how we relate to each other and how there may be internal conflict between different parts of ourselves. His entertaining accounts of transactional analysis are also useful to see how we bring mental representations of relationships to new situations.

Like Freud, Berne also postulated three parts to the mind, namely Parent (Superego) Adult (Ego) and Child (Id). He suggested a simplified version of mental representation of self and other in which we adopt a 'set' of behaviours which corresponds to a version of child, adult or parent, and expect another person to fulfil the complementary role. He postulated that any one of these three parts of the personality may be dominant at any time and will determine how we conduct a relationship or a transaction. The degree and nature of the emotion in the transaction will partly determine the chosen role.

If I take my car to the garage for a service this is probably an emotionally neutral transaction in which I have a business arrangement with the mechanic. This will be an Adult–Adult transaction.

I may consult my GP about a sore throat and feel calm and sensible: I want simple diagnosis and treatment. Another Adult–Adult transaction. If, however, I have vomited blood I may visit my GP feeling very frightened and helpless, desperately wanting her to sort it out for me. In my mind I feel again like a child needing my mother to fix things and turn to the GP to take control, perhaps attributing exaggerated ability to her. This would be a Child–Parent transaction.

I visit my tutor to tell him I am behind with my essay because I can't find the recommended references. I expect criticism and a lecture on laziness and I am pleasantly surprised to be treated like an adult and advised where to get what I need. I expected an unpleasant Child–Parent transaction and got an Adult–Adult one instead.

Once again it is clear that we bring certain expectations to new situations and new relationships, and that these are related to our existing mental representations. We will return to this concept of expected transactions when we think about the therapeutic relationship.

Freud's developmental theory: early determinants of personality and behaviour

MAIN POINTS

- Freud proposed that children's mental development proceeds in a series of stages corresponding to their bodily development.

- Freud's oral stage is in the first year, and corresponds to the time when the child uses its mouth a great deal for pleasure and to relate to the world.

- Freud's anal stage takes place in the second and third years and corresponds to the time when the child gains sphincter control and his interest is focused on this new skill.

- Freud's genital stage takes place in the third to fifth years and corresponds to the child's awareness of difference between the sexes, ability to find pleasure in his own genitals, and curiosity about other people's bodies.

The practice of psychoanalysis and psychodynamic psychotherapy have a strong developmental bias. That is, they work on the assumption that personality and behaviour are determined partly by innate, inherited factors, partly by the environment in which a person is brought up and overall on the way in which the interaction between these leads to representations of self and other in the mind.

Freud took a Darwinian view of human development and believed that aspects of infant behaviour were biologically programmed to ensure survival of the species. He considered that the infant drive for contact with other humans was biologically determined and a way to maximise behaviours which would ultimately lead to opportunities for sexual contact and thus propagation of the human species. It was this idea that human activity must somehow be directed towards species survival and therefore sexual activity which led to the misunderstanding that Freud interpreted everything in terms of sex.

In addition, Freud suggested that psychological development takes place in a series of developmental stages which correspond to the physical stages of children's development. He observed that the child is most aroused or excited by different parts of the body at different developmental times and that this arousal is likely to shape or at least influence the way that the child conceptualises other aspects of the world and his experiences. He thought that a child could become stuck or fixated at a particular stage, and that certain undesirable character traits would result.

Freud proposed three stages in the child's first five years.

1 The **oral stage** corresponds to the first year. During this time the child relates to the world to a large extent through his mouth, and gets a lot of pleasure from sucking and tasting. Freud thought that the child's mental process during this time was structured around images of feeding, and of taking things in and spitting them out. According to this way of thinking, a person fixated at this stage would show excessive dependency and demandingness or greed for other people.

2 The **anal stage** corresponds to the second and third years. During this time the child learns sphincter control and becomes capable of holding on to or expelling the contents of his rectum and

bladder. It is also the time when he learns to crawl and walk, and begins to be able to move independently away from his mother. Freud thought that issues in the child's mental development were independence and control. Fixation at this stage would lead to anxiety about control, including obsessional control, meanness and rigidity.

3 The **genital stage** corresponds to the third to fifth years. During this time the child becomes aware of his own and other people's gender and of his or her own genitals, which are also a source of pleasure. This is the stage at which Freud introduced the notion of the Oedipus complex.

The Oedipus complex

MAIN POINTS

- Children show a particular interest in their own and other people's sexuality at around 3–5 years. This interest is not confined to this time, however.

- They are aware that their parents have a relationship from which they are excluded. They may feel rivalrous with one or other parent.

- This developmental hurdle highlights important aspects of development, including the acceptance of difference, the limits to what one can be and can have, the necessity of tolerating being left out of others' relationships and the ability to be curious about one's own and other people's sexual activity.

- Later difficulties linked with this developmental stage include fear of rivalry, excessive anxiety about sexuality and fear of commitment to a sexual relationship.

Although children can identify themselves as male or female from about two years old, they often become particularly interested in their own and other people's genitals at about three to five years. They also have strong attachments to their parents and, for example, commonly declare their intention to marry a parent when they grow up. By this age the child is aware that his or her parents have a relationship from which he or she is excluded. In addition, by this time the child is confronted with the reality that as a boy he will grow up to be a man like his father or as a girl she will grow up to be a woman like her mother, and that however much the child wants it he or she cannot be biologically like the other parent.

The Oedipus complex has been somewhat revised since Freud's notoriously phallocentric version and is regarded by dynamic psychotherapists as centrally important in development. Most clinicians would not restrict this important maturational hurdle however to a period of two years between the ages of three and five, but assume that although it may be important at this stage in childhood, it will remain an issue throughout the child's development. Learning to negotiate a three-person relationship is a fundamental step for the child, not only in the early years but throughout life. The presence of an intact family is not essential for these issues to be relevant, although different family structures must modify the child's experience. The Oedipal stage is significant for the following reasons:

- The child realises that he or she is male or female and will grow up to be like one parent but not both. He or she has to resolve any resentment about not ever being able to have what the other sex has. It may be difficult for a little boy to accept that he cannot grow up to be a woman and have a baby, and for a little girl to accept that she will never have a penis and be a man.

- The child loves and desires both parents and is rivalrous with each for the other. Learning to accept that the parents have a special relationship from which he or she is excluded is painful. The resolution of this, however, forms the basis of learning to be left out of later situations, and also frees the child to separate from the parents (in adolescence) and find his or her own intimate relationships.

- The parents' relationship will itself have some mental representation in the child's mind and the quality of this will be affected by the actual state of the parents' affection and care for each other, and also by the fantasies which the child has about what they do together. Some children are alarmed by their own aggressive feelings and fantasies and may attribute these to the parents and what goes on between them in their sexual relationship.

- Fear of parental retaliation for their rivalrous wishes appears to be an issue for some children. A minority of children show signs of anxiety at around this age, which in most cases resolves without any therapeutic intervention.

Later difficulties suggested to relate to this stage of development include fear of competition or rivalry, anxiety about sexuality, fear of commitment to a sexual relationship and excessive anxiety or anger about being left out of relationships.

The present status of Freud's ideas

MAIN POINTS

- Some of Freud's ideas have been supported by later research.
- Some of his ideas have been discarded or modified in the light of new evidence.

A number of Freud's ideas have been borne out by developmental and neuropsychological research. The notion of unconscious mental process is not now disputed, and the idea of conflicting wishes leading to problems is widely accepted (Dixon and Henley, 1991). The term 'ego' is still employed, and tends to be used as Freud applied it, to the rational, reasonable part of the personality. 'Superego' is used to describe both a punitive part of the personality and conscience, the part which responds with guilt to wrongdoing. The term 'id' is now rarely used outside strictly psychoanalytic literature.

Freud's notion of the infant as a blank slate with instincts cannot now be accepted. There is good evidence from developmental research that the infant has a sense of its separate self from the start, and a strong need to develop relationships (Hobson, 1993). This need, the infant's ability to seek contact and the quality of available relationships largely determine how the infant's innate qualities will be expressed. Freud said little about the importance of the quality of infant care in the early years and this yawning gap has been filled by others, both psychoanalytic writers and developmentalists. His ideas about developmental stages remain plausible, although so much more goes on for the infant that their importance is no longer considered central. The Oedipus complex has stood the test of time, although somewhat modified from the original.

Theories of development are regarded as important in psychotherapy because psychoanalysis (and dynamic therapy) is a method that is structured on the view that what happened early on is likely to appear later in life and to be accessed through the therapeutic relationship. Some analytic writers (Freud and, to an extent, Klein) based many of their ideas on what they observed in the therapeutic relationship with adults, which suggests a leap from present to past mental structure which may or may not be justified. Others (for example, Donald Winnicott, Margaret Mahler, Anna Freud) observed children and drew conclusions from these observations.

The contribution of Melanie Klein

MAIN POINTS

- Klein proposed that the infant is born with innate destructive impulses and that these will colour his interaction with the environment.

- She thought that the infant had a sense of a separate self from the beginning of life.

- Klein also thought that the infant had a sense of the parental relationship during the first year of life.

continued ...

- She proposed two stages or positions in mental development: the paranoid schizoid position and the depressive position.

- She elaborated this to describe the mental mechanism of projective identification. This has been centrally important in later psychodynamic thinking.

Klein formulated several new ideas:

- She emphasised the place of innate destructive impulses in the child from the beginning of life. She proposed that the child's development is influenced not only by the environment which the parents provide, but by the infant's propensity to interpret and colour his environmental experience and his thinking with his own innate aggressive feelings. These are said to be primitive in the sense that they are unmodified by actual experience, and are assumed to be extreme and frightening.

- She suggested that the infant has a sense of self and other from the beginning of life. This is supported by later developmental research.

- She thought that the infant had a sense of the parental relationship from the first year, rather than the fourth or fifth year as Freud suggested. She derived this idea from her work with young children.

- She described the very young infant splitting his experience into good and bad. She called this stage of development the paranoid schizoid position. This would be consistent with later cognitive developmental research which indicates that an infant categorises experience from the beginning of its life. Klein also thought that the infant split his own mixed sensations into good and bad and projected one or the other into the outside world, so that his perceptions would then become coloured by whatever feelings he had projected. This would affect his relationship with the person who was the unwitting recipient of the projected feelings.

- She further suggested that during the first year the infant gradually learns that he can have good and bad feelings towards the same person. She called this the depressive position. This use of the word 'depressive' is not related to either the symptom of depression nor the diagnostic category of depression. It was called 'depressive' because she thought that the baby had some realisation that he could feel destructive feelings towards the mother whom he also loved, and that this would induce a feeling of sadness.

Klein has been criticised for imputing sophisticated thinking to infants at an early age. Whether or not one agrees with this in relation to infants, her ideas have been extremely useful in working with disturbed adult patients suffering from severe personality disorders, who habitually use the mental mechanisms of splitting and projection which she described. (See p. 75 for further discussion of projective mechanisms.)

Attachment theory and attachment behaviour

MAIN POINTS

- Attachment theory begins from a Darwinian position that humans are designed to show early behaviours which will promote survival. Infant behaviours which increase attachment are therefore adaptive in these terms.

- Humans need attachment figures throughout their life. Children need attachment figures for protection. Adults need them for contact and comfort.

- John Bowlby was first to identify attachment as a specific class of behaviour. His important early research with James Robertson in the 1950s was observation of children separated from parents in hospitals and residential care.

- Later research focused on assessing the quality of the security of attachment to the parent(s) and to classification of children's behaviour into secure and different patterns of insecure.

continued ...

- Security in children is relationship-specific. The child may be secure with one parent and insecure with the other.

- Security is suggested to relate to the parent's ability to empathise with the child's state of mind, especially when the child's attachment needs are aroused.

- An assessment of adult mental representation of attachment was developed in the mid-1980s. Adults, like children, can be classified into secure and insecure, though in adults the classifications are called autonomous and non-autonomous.

- There is a high correlation between a parent's attachment pattern and that of the child with him or her. The child's one-year security with that parent can be predicted with some confidence from assessing the parent during pregnancy.

- Classifications at one year have some predictive value for later psychosocial development. The child with two secure attachments does best; the child with two insecure attachments least well.

Attachment theory

John Bowlby construed child development rather differently from Freud or Klein (Bowlby, 1988). Bowlby was interested in Darwin's ideas about evolution and like Freud, thought that the primary motivational force for human behaviour was evolutionary and biological. However, where Freud thought that survival of the species was determined by behaviour which maximised sexual contact, Bowlby considered that behaviours which maximised the *survival* of the infant were important and were determined by evolution. Bowlby proposed that infant attachment to a care-giver was the optimal way to ensure survival of the human infant. The need for attachment was therefore not only central to the survival of the individual but also to survival of the species. According to this theory, much infant behaviour with the care-giver and much adult behaviour in intimate relationships relates to the human need for attachment.

The work begun by Bowlby has been influential both in psychotherapy and in developmental research. One of the strengths of this theory is that it allows for systematic behavioural observations as well as theoretical ideas about psychological development.

The attachment figure

Animals who are threatened or frightened seek a place of safety, a hole or a burrow; young animals often run to a parent. Children who are frightened or anxious use attachment figures as a source of protection and safety. Children usually have several attachment figures, but the child's overall sense of security is mainly determined by the quality of the relationship with the person who does most of the care. Adults depend on their attachment figures for contact, emotional and physical, and for comfort.

Situations in which a person feels anxious or threatened with pain or loss are likely to arouse attachment behaviour. This has implications for medical care.

The innate aspect of attachment

Infants are born with innate (genetically determined) characteristics which lead them to seek contact with other humans. For example, they have an inborn tendency to seek the shape of the human face, although they also soon learn by association to recognise the familiar features of the face. Like other young primates, they have an innate tendency to cling and follow their familiar care-giver. In the second half of the first year, these behaviours are organised into specific attachment behaviours to certain figures in the infant's life.

These specific attachment behaviours include proximity-seeking and contact maintenance. More variable behaviours are learned in the context of the quality of the relationship available to the infant. Thus in the optimal situation the infant will learn to expect that when his attachment needs are aroused, he can seek contact and comfort, and his care-giver will recognise his state of mind and respond appropriately. If for some reason the care-giver cannot provide this response reliably, the infant will develop some strategy for coping with his aroused attachment needs.

Early observation of attachment behaviour

In the early 1950s, John Bowlby and James and Joyce Robertson studied young children who were separated from their parents for a prolonged period. They made a series of video films of children in hospital and residential care (Robertson and Robertson, 1969). Their descriptions and film records of the distressing effect of long separation on young children had a considerable impact on the hospital management of children, and to some extent on other institutional child care. Where previously parents were discouraged from staying with their child in hospital, it is now considered good practice to have parents remain with a child who has to spend time in hospital.

Assessment of infant security of attachment

Systematic research from the late 1960s onwards began to look at attachment in more detail, and to examine the effect of quality of attachment on the child's development when there had not been long separations and the child had been cared for continuously by one or both parents.

Research has consistently shown that in the US and UK, about two-thirds of children are securely attached to their mothers and about one-third show some degree of insecurity. Secure children are confident that the mother will be a reliable source of protection and safety, while insecure children experience mother as a not entirely reliable source of protection and have to find some strategy to cope with this.

Infant security can be assessed at one year in a standardised test situation involving two brief separations from the mother and two

2dcp + 2reun   Mahler?

reunions (the Strange Situation). Three kinds of behaviour have been described:

1 secure

2 avoidant insecure

3 ambivalent insecure.

Secure infants welcome the mother even if they have been distressed by the separation; they do not show anger, they seek proximity and comfort, and soon return to play.

Insecure infants find their anxiety heightened by the uncertainty of maternal response to their distress and they deal with this in one of two ways:

1 One group ignores the mother's going away and ignores her return. If the mother makes an approach to the child it is avoided or treated with indifference. The child often shows more interest in the toys in the playroom than in the mother. This behaviour is called *avoidant insecure* behaviour.

2 The other group of insecure infants deal with their anxiety by showing an angry clinging to the mother. They often get very upset by her going away even for a minute, and on her return angrily demand contact but show resistance when they get it, are slow to settle with repeated outbursts of crying, and are reluctant to return to play. This is called *ambivalent insecure* behaviour.

It is important to realise that both these groups are showing a coherent strategy for dealing with a stressful situation. Infant insecurity has been linked to maternal insensitivity to the child's cues and signals. As a result, the child can never be sure that he will get the response he needs when he is upset. He may, for example, have a mother who simply does not notice or realise what her child needs, or a mother who needs her child to respond to her rather than the other way round. In using either avoidant or ambivalent behaviour, the child has learned a way to reduce his anxiety.

Correlation between early insecure behaviour and later development

It seems that secure attachment acts as a protective factor against the vicissitudes of life, and at five and 10 years secure children more easily make friends, are better liked by both peers and adults, and are more socially confident.

- Children who are insecure at one year have more difficulty than secure children in making friends when they go to school and are less liked by teachers.

- There is a slight delay in language and cognitive development in insecure children, but the principal effect is on social competence and confidence.

- Children rated as avoidant at one year show some tendency to bully other children at five and 10 years, while those rated as ambivalent may be victims of bullying and tend to be oversensitive and easily hurt.

- Secure children make fewer bids for a teacher's attention and are more likely to be attended. They seem to be good at getting the response they want.

- Secure children are better at resolving playground disputes. They either negotiate, or if that is not feasible, leave the dispute.

- If secure children of five or six years are shown a strip cartoon showing an ambiguous situation they will tend to attribute benign intent. *The boy accidentally knocked over the girl's toy.* Insecure children will tend to attribute malign intent. *The boy knocked over the girl's toy on purpose.*

- It has been suggested that secure children are more socially competent because they are more empathic than insecure children and they are therefore more skilled at sensing how other people feel and how they should be approached.

There are of course degrees of insecurity, some children are highly insecure, others on the boundary of secure/insecure. It must be recognised that security of attachment is only one factor which shapes the personality of the developing child.

Adult attachment

The assessment of adult attachment for research or clinical purposes is not made by observation of behaviour but by evaluating the mental representation of attachment in the adult. The assessment is made using an analysis of the transcript of a semi-structured interview in which the subject is asked a number of questions relating to early experience of attachment relationships. The evaluation depends not on a rating of actual or remembered experience, but on the degree to which the subject has been able to form a coherent narrative regarding his own attachment, *to recognise states of mind and motive in both self and attachment figures*, and to value attachment to others, even if his own experience was unsatisfactory.

About two-thirds of adults are classified as *autonomous* with respect to attachment, with an ability to be reasonably coherent about their attachment experience, to be aware of other people's states of mind when discussing attachment experiences and to value attachment relationships.

About 20% are *dismissing* of attachment, tending to idealise early relationships while being unable to offer evidence to support their idealisation. Despite the idealisation they are either overtly derogatory of attachment behaviour or apparently unaware of its relevance in relationships. They may be rather grandiose in their insistence that they do not need other people. The narrative is generally somewhat incoherent when attachment relationships are being described.

About 15% of people are *preoccupied* with respect to attachment. Although valuing of attachment, they have a sense of still being actively involved in early attachments, with little indication that they have resolved their feelings about these relationships, and often show continuing anger with early attachment figures. Like dismissing individuals, they are not very coherent in their account of attachment relationships.

A person can be very coherent in discussing other matters, but still be incoherent when talking about attachment. It appears that the continuing anxiety about attachment is associated with a degree of inability to think and speak clearly about attachment relationships.

The concept of self-reflection

The care-giver's (generally the parent) capacity to reflect on her own and other people's state of mind when attachment needs are aroused correlates highly with infant security. Adults who are relatively non-anxious about their own attachment relationships can attribute intentions and meanings to their own and other people's behaviour in situations where they need or seek attachment. Adults who remain anxious about attachment become relatively incoherent in describing their close relationships, and in particular have difficulty in conceptualising *why* the people concerned behave as they do (Fonagy and Target, 1997).

Intergenerational transmission of attachment

There is a high correlation between the parental representation of attachment and the child's attachment behaviour at one year. By assessing a parent in pregnancy, it is possible to predict with 70–80% certainty what the attachment pattern of the child will be with the parent at one year. An autonomous parent is likely to have a child who is secure with her or him, a dismissing parent a child who is avoidantly insecure with her or him and a preoccupied parent a child who is ambivalently insecure with her or him (Fonagy *et al.*, 1991).

The measure of infant security is *relationship-specific*. The child may be secure with one parent and insecure with the other, depending on the quality of the parent's representation of attachment. The effect on the child's subsequent development is additive, in that the child does best if he has a secure relationship with both parents, and worst if he has an insecure relationship with both parents. The primary care-giver (usually mother) has the greater effect on the child's development in this respect.

The child's behaviour in the mildly stressful test situation leads to the arousal of his attachment needs. Insecure children will show defensive manoeuvres to deal with this. It seems that defensive or coping strategies are learned from parents by children by as early as the end of the first year.

Psychological defence mechanisms

MAIN POINTS

- We all have experiences in life which cause us painful emotion. We also have wishes which conflict with our rational or moral standards.

- People adopt various mental defence mechanisms to avoid mental pain or conflict.

- Defence mechanisms protect us from anxiety and other painful emotions: they are a way of reducing painful emotion.

- Defence mechanisms can be on a spectrum from conscious to unconscious.

- Everyone uses defences, both conscious and unconscious, and they are not necessarily pathological.

- The end product of the mechanisms may be a form of maladaptive behaviour or a neurotic symptom. If there is an underlying wish the symptom may express the original wish in disguised form.

We are all subject to feelings and thoughts which cause us distress. This sense of distress includes feelings of fear or anxiety, shame, guilt and perhaps an acute sense of loss. These may be caused by something in the external world, for example I may be distressed by the thought of having a serious illness and the underlying fear that I may not survive or may be seriously disabled.

They may be because of something internal, something which is already in my mind. This may be a thought or wish which conflicts with my self-image or with the moral standards I want to adhere to. A thought or memory which lowers my self-esteem may make me feel ashamed or guilty. Or I may be distressed because I have thoughts and feelings which I find abhorrent, for example violent or sexual wishes which conflict with my moral standards.

Most, though not all, of these experiences of mental discomfort have a component of anxiety. Anxiety is a useful signal to us that we are in some way endangered and that we should take avoiding action. This is clearly not always possible, so we must either tolerate the uncomfortable feeling or find some other way of reducing it.

We find ways of reducing unwanted feelings either consciously or unconsciously. Conscious ways of reducing unwanted feelings may be adaptive or maladaptive. For example, if I am anxious about an exam I am sitting in two weeks and for which I have done no work, I can avoid anxiety by suppressing any thoughts of the exam and diverting myself with an active social life, or I can reduce anxiety by studying for the exam. Arguably one solution is more adaptive than the other.

Unconscious ways of reducing anxiety or other painful feelings may also be adaptive or maladaptive. For example, a person may function well at least for a time, by being able to unconsciously deny some of his own needs and throw himself into work. On the other hand, at another time this may become maladaptive if it leads to overwork and breakdown.

Definition

Defence mechanisms are mental or behavioural strategies which reduce anxiety or other painful affects.

Characteristics of mental defence mechanisms

- Defence mechanisms reduce anxiety or other painful affect.
- They can be conscious or unconscious.
- Everyone uses them in everyday life.
- They can be adaptive or maladaptive, pathological or helpful.

- Sometimes symptoms are the result of defensive mechanisms to avoid unwanted feelings.

- The underlying wish that leads to anxiety may be expressed in the defensive solution.

Case example

A senior nurse was devoted to her work and to her patients. She worked long hours, often staying well beyond her shift to be with a distressed patient. She had a reputation for being the kind of nurse who could never do too much for her patients. She led a quiet, rather lonely life outside work, but got such satisfaction from nursing that she felt her life was comfortable. Her health was good until she contracted glandular fever, which was followed by a prolonged depression which required hospital admission. During the admission she was a most demanding patient, often exhausting and exasperating the staff with her demands for attention and support.

She had dealt with her own unconscious wish for attention and care by denying it in herself, splitting it off from her own self-image and projecting it on to her sick and vulnerable patients. She was able to satisfy her own need vicariously by caring for her patients with great devotion. When she was ill herself, however, and feeling helpless and unable to look after other people, her usual defence mechanism was not available to her and her own need was more directly expressed.

She had in fact found quite an adaptive way of dealing with a side of herself which could perhaps never be satisfied in personal relationships. The problem with such an adaptation (or defence) is its tendency to break down when external circumstances change, as it did in this case.

When she was admitted to hospital her own strong wish to be looked after, previously repressed and unconscious, became conscious. She might have dealt with this new awareness by talking about how unhappy she felt and working out what this might have to do with her early life experiences. This would have been very painful and she would have had to acknowledge to herself her acute sense of deprivation and her sadness that she could never have the kind of childhood care that she longed for. She would also have had to accept that she would need to find some other solution to this need which could never be met as she longed for it to be.

Her solution in hospital was to regress to a state of childish neediness and to make the unreasonable demands on her carers that a small child might reasonably make on a parent. Not surprisingly these could not be met. A temporary regression may be very helpful in allowing a physically or mentally ill person to get care and support to recover from the illness; a longer-term regression is generally unhelpful because it stops the person from managing their usual ways of coping with life's difficulties.

Common defence mechanisms

Repression

Two businessmen are dining with an important visitor. During the meal the conversation turns to schools and the visitor says that he has just taken his son to school in ——shire. 'Oh my neighbour has a kid at school in ——shire,' says one of the hosts, 'but it's a school for loopy kids, his son has Down's syndrome.' 'The same school no doubt,' says the visitor coldly, 'my son is handicapped.'

A year later, over drinks, his colleague reminds him of this appalling faux pas – he has absolutely no memory of it.

He has *repressed* this painful moment of acute embarrassment, and need not experience the anxiety which the memory would arouse.

Reaction formation

Aggression is something many people regard as 'bad' in themselves. It is also part of normal experience. So how can a person deal with his unacceptable wish to be aggressive? Perhaps by using it to destroy anything which is tainted with aggression. An aggressive person may become a determined pacifist (though of course not all pacifists repress aggressive feelings). He can then fight for the cause of pacifism and in doing so satisfy his aggressive drives.

This mechanism which both gratifies and repudiates an unac-ceptable drive is called *reaction formation*.

Mrs Grey spent a lot of time writing to television companies to complain about programmes with unacceptable scenes of explicit sexual behaviour. She also spent time searching the newspapers and watching television so that she could spot these threats to public morality.

Denial

Denial is the mechanism whereby in the face of all logical evidence a person behaves as though reality is not happening.

A patient was found to have a potentially fatal illness. His diagnosis was explained to him by the consultant who invited him to bring his wife for further discussion. The patient arrived for the appointment alone and had no memory that his wife was invited. A week into treatment the wife demanded a meeting with the consultant and was horrified to hear the diagnosis which she (and later the patient) denied any knowledge of. She sent a formal complaint to the hospital.

The patient was so frightened by the diagnosis that he denied to himself that he had heard it. The process was unconscious. Denial is different from repression in that it involves some obliteration of current reality.

Rationalisation

Rationalisation occurs when an external agency is held to be responsible for an internal event.

I failed my viva because he asked all the wrong questions.

The woman who says 'I'm depressed because people don't like me' is trying to make sense of or *rationalise* her inexplicable depression.

Her observation may be accurate, but she may find it difficult to see that there may be something in her attitude to people which makes them avoid her.

Projective identification

This mental mechanism was first described by Melanie Klein (see above). She proposed that small children tend to see things in black-and-white terms, and assume that a thing or a person is either entirely good or entirely bad. She called this *splitting*. As the child gets older, he begins to realise that this is not how the world is, and becomes increasingly able to accommodate the idea that people are both good and bad and that he can have good and bad feelings towards the same person. However, we never entirely lose our tendency to split the world into good and bad. Articles in the tabloid press may demonstrate the mechanisms of splitting.

In times of stress, we are especially prone to *split* within ourselves, to *deny* the part that is unacceptable and to externalise it and attribute it to (or *project* it into) someone or something outside ourselves. This triad of *splitting*, *denial* and *projection* is a universal mental mechanism and of central importance in understanding how people relate to each other.

Thus the nurse (see above) *denied* her own vulnerability, *split* it off from conscious awareness and *projected* her unwanted needy feelings into her patients. It is not unknown for doctors to do this too. This mechanism in medical practice may lead to the kind of devoted care described for the nurse, who did not despise her own vulnerability, but unconsciously wanted it to be caringly responded to.

In contrast to this, some people dislike their own need for care which they find humiliating. Like the nurse they project it into other people, but unlike her they then treat it and the other person patronisingly or even contemptuously. This mechanism probably lies behind the 'arrogance' that patients sometimes complain of in their doctors.

The therapeutic relationship: working alliance, transference and countertransference

MAIN POINTS

- We bring our mental representations or working models of self and others to new relationships and new situations.

- These lead us to have expectations of how another person will behave and feel in the relationship.

- We give verbal and non-verbal cues which invite the behaviours we expect.

- The therapeutic relationship in psychodynamic psychotherapy is actively used so that the patient's mental representations can be played out and analysed in a safe setting.

- The therapeutic relationship has three components: the working alliance, transference and countertransference.

- The working alliance is the business contract which allows the work to take place.

- The transference is the unconscious process by which the patient's mental representations of expected behaviour are attributed to the therapist, who is experienced and treated as a figure in the patient's inner world.

- The countertransference is the feelings which the therapist has towards the patient, some of which will relate to the therapist's own mental models and experience, and some of which will be elicited by the patient's projected expectations.

- Therapists have personal therapy to be more aware of their mental models so that these contaminate the therapeutic relationship as little as possible.

We bring our existing mental representations of the world and ourselves to new relationships. These representations may be thought of as a range of scenarios or stories with self and another person or people, each with some emotion attached. This is our prototype or working model for approaching new situations, where we will tend to use old information to give us rules about how to deal with it. We project our internal images or expectations into the new relationship and expect to find a familiar response.

In addition, we not only expect a particular response, but unconsciously may actually try to elicit it by giving verbal and non-verbal messages which invite another person to behave as we expect.

Example: *Rob grew up feeling that he could never satisfy his parents. He felt that they had high expectations of their children and he believed that he was a disappointment to them. He was shy and uncertain when he went to school and was bullied by some of the other children. As a rather isolated student, he forced himself to go to a party, hoping he would make friends and have a better social life. He went into the party stiff with anxiety, did not make eye contact with anyone and stood alone looking miserable and tense. His body language told people that he was afraid of contact and that he feared being disappointing, and the students at the party responded as he expected and did not approach him. He left feeling he had been rejected just as he had dreaded, but did not realise how much he had invited the feared response.*

Rob has an (unconscious) internal representation of himself with other people in which he is unable to give people what they want and is rejected because he disappoints them. Although he knows rationally that he must try to make friends if his life is to be happier, he unconsciously sabotages his own efforts by giving messages to other people that he expects the relationship to fail.

How can we help a person access and understand the unconscious mental representations which hold them back from sorting out emotional problems? There are two kinds of psychotherapy which try to get access to the patient's representational world. Cognitive psychotherapy explores the conscious and almost conscious thoughts underlying maladaptive behaviour. Psychodynamic psychotherapy also explores these thoughts, but in addition attempts to help the patient to find the unconscious beliefs and assumptions which underlie his maladaptive behaviours and feelings.

More than any other kind of psychotherapy, psychodynamic psychotherapy makes very active use of the relationship between patient and therapist as part of the therapeutic process. It is within this relationship that the patient will be able to enact at least some of what he cannot remember or cannot bring to his conscious thinking. The therapist is constantly alert, and closely observes not only the patient's overt behaviour, but also the quality of the relationship which he creates in the therapy.

There are three parts to the therapeutic relationship in psychodynamic psychotherapy:

1 the working alliance (also called the therapeutic alliance)

2 the transference

3 the countertransference.

The working alliance

Definition: The *working alliance* is the agreement between patient and therapist that they will work together on the patient's emotional or psychological problems. It is a contractual arrangement and is a rational and adult transaction.

Any contract between a doctor and patient requires an agreement. In some situations the patient's cooperation is less important than in others. If a patient is brought in unconscious to the Accident & Emergency department his immediate cooperation is not relevant to the treatment. If a patient is admitted for an operation, he has to cooperate to agree to have the operation, to come on the agreed day and to fast on the morning he goes to theatre. In some ways, however, he is a relatively passive recipient of the treatment. The surgical team will act upon his body to produce the required changes.

A greater degree of cooperation is needed for a patient to have psychotherapy. The treatment requires the patient's active involvement to work over a period of weeks, months or even years. Some patients are unable or unwilling to enter into such an agreement, which needs a commitment to regular attendance, a willingness to explore one's own behaviour and to tolerate sometimes painful thoughts, feelings and memories.

The transference

Definition: *Transference* is the transferring of feelings which belong to a relationship from the past into a present relationship. This process is unconscious. The attributions are inappropriate to the present relationship.

When a patient enters into a regular therapeutic relationship with a therapist he is likely to develop a degree of attachment to the therapist and to feel some dependency on this person who listens non-judgementally and who is interested in his story and relationships. It is an unusual relationship, which is both intimate and professional. Although the therapist learns a great deal about the patient, she does not give personal information in return, and this imbalance allows the patient to imagine and assume what he chooses about the therapist. In doing so the patient has to use his own mental images and expectations.

This is similar to the situation described above when the young man, Rob, went to a party with expectations which were almost inevitably fulfilled. We expect our patients to bring their mental images and internal relationships into the therapeutic relationship and to project some of them on to the therapist, who unlike Rob's classmates will not enact them but will try to clarify them for the patient. In this setting, unconscious expectations can be elucidated and understood.

While no one at Rob's party was likely to explain to him how his mental model was wrecking his behaviour, this is precisely what we do expect to happen in psychotherapy. The therapist pays close attention to the behavioural and verbal hints about what the patient's assumptions and unconscious expectations are, and together therapist and patient work out what is going on under the surface. This central therapeutic activity of psychodynamic psychotherapy is called the analysis of the transference relationship.

The countertransference

Definition: *Countertransference* is the feeling or feelings elicited in the therapist by the patient's behaviour and communications.

The setting for the therapy is intended to facilitate the patient recreating his inner world in the therapy and bringing his expectations of relationships to the therapeutic relationship. All doctors and all therapists have feelings about their patients, but in this particular setting the therapist's feelings are important in helping to understand something of what is going on in the patient's mind.

One of the therapist's tasks is to identify the responses the patient generates in her by the patient projecting something of his mental representations, i.e. in the transference relationship.

Example: *Mr Green had a childhood history of rather unavailable parents and inconsistent parental care. He reported his father as a rather distant figure more interested in his work than the family. His mother had repeated episodes of severe depression, leaving Mr Green and his older brother to fend for themselves. As an adult, he himself had had spells of depression which did not respond well to antidepressant treatment. He reported short-lived and unsatisfactory close relationships with women. In therapy, the therapist became aware that although he talked fluently about himself and his life, she felt rather distant and even a little bored. As there was no obvious reason for this feeling, she surmised that Mr Green was creating this sense of distance between them. As the therapy progressed and further work was done, it became clear that he was afraid to burden the therapist with his emotional state, and in particular his depressed feelings, just as he had been afraid to burden his emotionally fragile mother.*

The therapist got a clue to how Mr Green related to people whom he might want to depend on by being alert to the response which he evoked in her. As Mr Green became aware of this himself, he could see that he held people at a distance in other relationships because of the same fear. He was able to recognise that this fear was no longer appropriate to his life.

It is important that the therapist is as aware as she can be about her own unconscious expectations, so that she is in touch with her personal tendencies to make assumptions. This is one reason that dynamic psychotherapists are expected to have their own personal therapy or analysis before treating patients. If this is not practicable (for example, trainees in psychiatry are required to treat patients in dynamic psychotherapy, but are not always able or willing to have personal therapy) they should have supervision from an experienced psychotherapist.

Other psychoanalytic terms used in psychodynamic psychotherapy

MAIN POINTS

- Several terms commonly used in psychodynamic psychotherapy are explained.

- Enactment is the playing out within the therapy of mental representation which cannot be expressed verbally.

- Repetition compulsion is the tendency to repeat instead of remembering.

- Acting out is enactment which takes place outside the safer confines of the therapeutic relationship. It is usually damaging for the patient.

Enactment

Enactment is the term used to describe the playing out of a mental scenario rather than verbally describing the associated thoughts and feelings. To some degree this is an inevitable part of dynamic therapy. An important principle of psychodynamic therapy is that, to an extent, old relationships are recreated in therapy so that the patient can use his adult mind to step back and think about what is going on. In some kinds of therapy, regression or dependency is discouraged; in psychodynamic therapy it is temporarily encouraged so that it can be re-experienced and understood in the safe setting of the therapeutic relationship.

Case example

Ms Black begins therapy because of depression related to difficulty in main-taining relationships. She attributes this to her poor choice of partners. She is in her late twenties and is a graduate with a good job which she does well. She married after leaving university, to a man who had been a fellow student, but the marriage broke down about a year later. She was and is able to manage her life very competently in those aspects where relation-ships are not too intimate, but her history reveals that love affairs have been stormy and short-lived.

A few months into therapy she became demanding and emotionally fragile, oscillating between tearfully wanting understanding from the therapist and furiously accusing him of neglect and of deliberately dis-appointing her. Her conscious wish for a supportive and loving relation-ship was swamped by unconscious needs which she neither recognised nor understood. Consciously she saw and experienced herself as a highly capable, warm person who had been the victim of unreasonable partners.

Ms Black had spent much of her earliest years in hospital suffering from a chronic condition which improved in mid-childhood. Because of the distance from her home her family visited only rarely. She remarked that she had adapted so well that by the time she was four the nurses called her 'the extra little nurse'. When she returned to the family at the age of nine her parents had separated and her mother was only too glad to have a dependable eldest child to help her. The patient was responsible for the care of her younger siblings from mid-childhood and had been unfailingly supportive of her mother. Problems only arose in her adult life when she got into a relationship where she had a chance of being looked after. Then all her old childhood longings for care and support, long suppressed, were aroused, and she became impossibly demanding, angry and tearful when her partner would not or could not respond to her needs. She herself recognised that she was 'emotional' in her relationships, but perceived her partners as cold and withholding.

The therapy became an opportunity for her to reassess both her own behaviour and the needs which lay behind them. The therapist's ability to be reliably available and not to respond with anger or exasperation made her feel responded to and helped her to think more calmly about herself. Ms Black longed to recreate a relationship with a parental figure who would look after her as she would have liked to be looked after as a child. In the therapy she was able to see how her strong childhood feelings were actually damaging her adult relationships and she was able to have more conscious control over her life.

Repetition compulsion

Repetition compulsion is a term which derives from Freud's notion of the compulsion to repeat instead of remembering. Ms Black was demonstrating repetition compulsion in her relationships with partners, where she enacted her emotional need and her anger that she had not been responded to *without remembering* what this need or anger was originally about. When she made sense of her feelings of longing for care, she could remember or at least realise that she had wanted that care as a child, but because there was no chance of getting it she had resolved the situation by caring for others. As an adult, the trigger of a close relationship led to her being 'obliged to repeat' the child's insistent demand for affection, unconsciously attempting to get what she had not felt was adequate when she was a child. She could not recover and have less demanding relationships until she could consciously acknowledge her childhood deprivation and give up the hope that she could still get what was missing in childhood. Once she could mourn what she had missed, she was freed to form more realistic adult relationships.

Note that repetition compulsion is not the same as compulsive symptoms such as hand-washing seen in obsessive compulsive disorder. Hand washing in OCD can be considered as an expression of extreme anxiety about getting rid of the damaging effects of germs. This fear about something damaging or destructive is arguably a projection of anxiety about the subject's own feared impulses to damage. The most effective treatment is behavioural.

Acting out

Acting out is enactment which takes place outside therapy. A patient may have strong feelings stirred up in his therapy. Instead of containing them until he can explore them with the therapist he acts them out in another setting. This is sometimes destructive for the patient, and must be urgently addressed in the therapy. If the patient is really unable to contain certain emotional issues within the treatment setting it may be better for the patient to end the therapy.

Example: *Unlike Ms Black, Mr White who had similar relationship problems to Ms Black, did not allow his need for attention and affection to surface in the therapy. When there was a break in therapy Mr White became furiously angry and abusive towards his wife. He felt that she had lost interest in him and was giving all her time to the children. When he started his therapy again he realised that these were feelings he had towards the therapist who had left him to go on holiday. He had acted out feelings which were stirred up by the therapy in the outside world.*

Note that 'acting out' has nothing to do with drama therapy. It is not a therapeutic activity and is generally unhelpful for the patient.

A dynamic formulation of psychiatric diagnoses

MAIN POINTS

- A dynamic formulation suggests a personal meaning for a person's symptoms or behaviour.

- It is important not to generalise about the meaning of symptoms based on diagnostic classifications.

- However, some dynamics are commonly associated with particular symptoms.

- Some dynamic ideas are outlined for common psychiatric problems.

I have hesitated in writing this section because it is important not to generalise about the meaning of specific symptoms and it is essential to look at a particular person's problems and his individual thoughts, feelings and experience. Each person's illness occurs against the background of his personality and the life experience that has shaped him. It must also be remembered that for some patients there is a strong genetic component and/or important biological contribution to their illness or condition, and that the dynamic understanding may be of secondary importance. However, I realise that exam candidates are often asked to comment on the dynamics of a particular condition, so with that caveat, I hope these formulations may be useful.

A psychodynamic approach recognises and emphasises individual differences in the meaning of people's behaviours, but there are also certain dynamics which are commonly seen in relation to particular diagnostic groups. This section gives an outline of dynamics which are often encountered in people suffering from specific mental disorders.

A dynamic formulation suggests a personal meaning of a person's symptoms in terms of his or her psychological organisation. Even when the person is unlikely to benefit from a formal psychodynamic treatment, an understanding of the psychological reasons behind symptoms and clinical presentation may help a psychiatric team to plan treatment and may improve cooperation between patient and team because the patient feels that his individual feelings and problems are recognised and understood.

The conditions whose dynamics are outlined in this section include:

- depressive disorder

- mania and hypomania

- schizophrenia

- anxiety: anxiety states, post-traumatic stress disorders and phobias

- obsessive compulsive disorder and obsessional behaviour

- addictive behaviour

- eating disorders: anorexia nervosa and bulimia nervosa

- borderline personality disorder
- narcissistic personality disorder.

Depressive disorder

It is important to distinguish depressed mood from sadness. Depression is a much more complex emotion and includes sadness and anger and sometimes also guilt and shame. A person suffering from depressive disorder feels helpless and often has strong feelings of self-blame or worthlessness. He feels unloved and unlovable. He may hate himself so much that he feels he would be better dead. He may also feel angry that those closest to him have not been able to support and help him.

Common dynamics include:

- a denial of sadness, with anger turned against the self
- a sense of helplessness to carry out normal activities
- anger towards others.

A denial of sadness, with anger turned against the self

Many episodes of depressive disorder are precipitated by an identifiable external event. This is often a loss or disappointment which may be trivial but which may trigger by association memories of previous loss, or an awareness of the person's helplessness to control loss of people and things that really matter. The pain of loss, however, does not lead to acceptance and healthy mourning, but to *denial* of sadness, and in its place a feeling of anger. According to Freud in his paper *Mourning and melancholia*, the person *denies* the reality of loss and keeps the lost object (person) alive by *identification*. Anger felt towards the lost object is then turned on the self, now identified with the lost person. The depressed person accuses himself of failure, and of being a worthless person.

A sense of helplessness

A sense of loss brings with it a feeling of helplessness to prevent the loss of what we need and love. If the true sense of loss is denied and mourning does not take place, the feeling of helplessness may be *displaced* from its original source to other aspects of the person's life. Thus he may be unable to carry out activities which are well within his capacity.

Anger towards others

The anger which is felt towards the lost object is *displaced* on to a person or people in the present life of the depressed person. Hostility may be unconscious, but expressed in various aspects of behaviour, for example in making heavy demands on family or professionals, while at the same time apologising for being 'a nuisance'.

Mania and hypomania

In dynamic terms, mania is usually considered to be a defence against depression. There is a *denial* of depression or of the sense of helplessness associated with depression. The feeling of omnipotence and the grandiose behaviour often found in mania and hypomania are expressions of this denial. This is not to say that there is not neurochemical change, and most psychiatrists would consider it important to treat hypomania with drug therapy at least in the acute phase of the illness.

A less extreme presentation of manic behaviour is also seen in people who have narcissistic personality disorder. A dynamic understanding of manic behaviour is valuable in understanding these patients, where there is denial of depression and helplessness and the expression of grandiose ideas without the appearance of psychotic symptoms.

Schizophrenia

Like a person with a neurotic problem, the psychotic person may see the external world in terms of his own internal world but to a degree which is outside normal experience. His current perceptions may be interpreted as though part of his internal model. He loses the ability to distinguish between internal and external reality, between his own thoughts and events in the outside world.

Aspects of his internal world are *split* off and *projected* into the outside world in a very concrete way. Thus for example, an auditory hallucination which is a critical commentary on his behaviour may be considered in dynamic terms to be a self-criticism projected into an outside agency. A delusion that his thoughts can be read or that others can put thoughts into his mind may express his feeling that he has no privacy and no control over his own mind. His sense of the boundary of his self is fragmented and his subjective feeling that others can put things into his mind and take things out at will is expressed as a delusional belief.

Anxiety

Anxiety states

Anxiety is a normal and healthy response to perceived threat. Anxiety is considered to be pathological when the anxiety is out of proportion to any identifiable threat, or when the person cannot limit or regulate the anxiety in a manageable way.

People may be habitually anxious because they constantly expect something damaging to happen to them or to another person. This may be linked to an unconscious fantasy of the person's own destructiveness, which has to be controlled, or to a fear of that same destructiveness *projected* into the outside world and constantly guarded against.

Post-traumatic stress disorder

In post-traumatic stress disorder the excessive anxiety can be traced back to a real experience of overwhelming fear or threat. The person may or may not already have a sense of anxiety about his own destructive capacity but this can be augmented by the actual experience of a severe threat to life in the outside world. The real experience then confirms pre-existing fears or anxieties about the dangerousness of the world.

Specific phobias

It is assumed that there has been *displacement* of anxiety from one feared object to an associated one, possibly from an unconscious fear which cannot be controlled to a conscious and therefore potentially avoidable one.

Obsessive compulsive disorder and obsessional behaviour

Obsessive compulsive disorder

The person with OCD has an anxiety about unconscious wishes or impulses which are unacceptable to him and which are felt to be damaging to himself or to other people. These are usually to do with either hostile or sexual feelings.

The damaging wish is *projected* into something in the outside world, for example into dirt, which is experienced as dangerous. The person then feels intense anxiety about contact with this feared contaminant, which is *magically controlled* by certain rituals, such as washing a specific number of times.

Obsessional behaviour

As a personality characteristic, the obsessional wish for order and cleanliness may be considered to be a *reaction formation* to the wish to make a mess, perhaps a sexual or aggressive mess. The obsessional person is characteristically rather controlling of himself and others, and may be careful to the point of meanness. As a personality trait it can be positive if not too extreme.

Addictive behaviour

Common dynamics include:

- control of someone/something the person depends on
- fear that another person can ever cope with his needs
- anaesthetising painful feelings
- attacking or punishing another person.

Controlling a needed thing or person

In infancy, the baby is allowed the illusion that the people he needs and cares about are under his control. As the child gets older he gradually learns that love and attention have to be earned and that his parents and others have their own needs and have interests which exclude him.

Coming to terms with the fact that the people we most care about are separate and largely outside our control is part of the process of growing up. We learn that mature relationships involve a degree of independence as well as closeness to another person. People with low self-esteem are particularly vulnerable because they fear not only being disappointed, but expect that they will disappoint the person they care about.

One way to deny the pain of being separate and not being in control over a needed person is to use a substance as a substitute for a person. The defence mechanisms used are *denial* of dependence and *displacement* of the need from a person to a substance. Whereas a person cannot be picked up and dropped at will, and is not endlessly available, a bottle of alcohol or a dose of a pleasurable drug can be controlled in terms of both access and quantity. The person has the comfort of putting the pleasurable substance into his body without having to consider another person's needs and without the fear of the relationship being taken away.

Fear that no one can ever cope with his needs

Some people despair that their needs for attention and care can ever be met. Alcohol or drugs may then be used as a substitute for a loving relationship. The need is *displaced* from a person to a substance.

Anaesthetising painful feelings

A person who is depressed, fearful, anxious or angry may use alcohol or an addictive drug as a way of cutting off feelings. In the longer term it is not usually successful, as the same feelings are likely still to be there or even intensified when the effects of the alcohol or the drug have worn off. The defence mechanism used is *avoidance*.

Punishing someone else

Sometimes the addiction is obviously a way of punishing a partner or parent who can be hurt by the addictive behaviour. The addicted person may feel for example that his partner is not giving him the attention he needs, so turns to an addictive substance partly for gratification and partly to 'show' his partner that she has failed him. This may be a fully conscious process or there may be unconscious *denial* of hostility to the other person but enactment of it in the damaging behaviour.

Eating disorders

Anorexia nervosa

Common dynamics include:

- control of a body which feels out of control

- denial of anxiety about the dangerous level of starvation and a sense of triumph over bodily needs
- denial of the reality of an adult sexual body.

Control of a body which feels out of control

The adolescent suffering from anorexia nervosa is often conflicted about separating from her parents, both longing for the closeness of a small child and her parent, and at the same time fearing that such closeness will lead to a loss of identity.

The onset of puberty with the bodily changes of an adult sexual body signals a process which will lead to separation from the family, and the demands of seeking close relationships elsewhere. At the same time the hormonal changes of puberty lead to states of arousal and a biologically driven impulse for physical intimacy. This is alarming for the adolescent who feels herself to be out of control and fears that her bodily needs will push her towards either a regressive intimacy with a parent or a relationship outside the family for which she is not ready.

Starvation becomes a solution which allows both suppression of sexual arousal and the recovery of a child-like body which will not signal sexual maturity to other people.

Denial of anxiety about the dangerous level of starvation and a sense of triumph over bodily needs

The patient usually shows no anxiety about the danger she is putting herself in. Instead there is often a *denial of the helplessness she feels in her body's sexual development* and a *manic triumph* in the way she is able to control her bodily needs. Anxiety and a sense of helplessness are *projected* into family and those who are treating her, who find themselves feeling all the frustration and worry relating to the situation.

Denial of the reality of an adult sexual body

It has been the author's clinical experience that some women with anorexia nervosa who recover normal weight may then behave as though their bodies were still child-shaped and may dress or otherwise behave in a socially inappropriate way. The reality of what it means to have a sexually mature body and how this affects other people may be *denied*.

Bulimia nervosa

Some people who suffer from eating disorder alternate between symptoms of anorexia and of bulimia. Others have either only anorexic or only bulimic symptoms.

People who compulsively binge and vomit may long for intimacy, but at the same time be afraid of it. There is a simultaneous belief that intimacy damages but is intensely desirable. Thus when closeness is possible the bulimic person gets panicky that something damaging will happen either to her or to the other person.

There is often a chronic feeling of emotional deprivation and emptiness which she seeks to fill in her frantic need for large quantities of food. The sense of deprivation is *displaced* from a person to food, a controllable object. As soon as the food is safe inside, however, she becomes anxious that it will damage her and she has to get rid of it quickly. Thus she controls her needed object by being able to take it in, very much as the alcoholic does, but unlike the alcoholic she further controls by expelling it. Vomiting is often followed by a sense of relief and euphoria, which may have components of both a chemical response to changes in blood sugar and a psychological 'high' (*manic denial* of helplessness and feeling of omnipotent control).

Borderline personality disorder

There is a characteristic constellation of anxieties which include several described above in people with anxiety or eating disorder and those who use addictive substances for self-calming. The person with borderline personality disorder longs for closeness but is frightened of the damage that can occur between people, so panics when a close relationship begins to develop. There is characteristically a pattern of clinging and demandingness in relationships followed by abrupt withdrawal. There is great difficulty in self-calming, so that distress is not quickly followed by a useful defensive activity, but by escalating arousal and a sense of disintegration. The panic may be expressed in an outburst of rage or in some physical activity which re-establishes a sense of contact with the world and a feeling of greater control. These may include self-cutting, bingeing or substance abuse.

There is a rigid view of self and the world and the person can become acutely upset if the world does not match the expectations which are projected on to it. For example, self-esteem is precarious and there may be an apparent self-confidence which quickly disintegrates when feedback from others does not confirm the image. The person will then rapidly fall into acute distress.

Narcissistic personality disorder

The narcissistic defences of grandiosity and arrogance are sometimes seen in people who have a borderline personality. The level of social functioning is usually better than for those with borderline personality and someone with a narcissistic personality may function fairly well, especially in non-intimate relationships, such as at work. Like people with borderline personality, however, they are acutely sensitive to slights and easily feel humiliated and diminished. Their self-esteem is precarious and they are vulnerable to sudden plunges of mood following a disappointment or a real or imagined criticism. Lesser degrees of narcissistic personality traits are common and may be compatible with a high level of competence at work, along with vulnerability in personal relationships, especially where the person has to be emotionally dependent on someone else. Dependence of another person is felt as humiliating and 'intimate' relationships may be tolerated only by aloofness and distancing. The emotional needs of other people may be defensively regarded with contempt, which can be acutely painful for a partner.

References

Bowlby J (1979) *The Making and Breaking of Affectional Bonds.* Tavistock, London.

Dixon N and Henley S (1991) Unconscious perception: possible implications of data from academic research for clinical practice. *Journal of Nervous and Mental Disorders.* **79**: 243–51.

Fonagy P, Steele M and Steele H (1991) Maternal representations of attachment during pregnancy predict the organisation of mother–infant attachment at one year of age. *Child Development.* **62**: 891–905.

Fonagy P and Target M (1997) Attachment and self-reflective function: their role in self-organisation. *Development and Psychopathology.* **9**(4): 679–700.

Hobson RP (1993) *Autism and the Development of Mind.* Lawrence Erlbaum, Hillsdale, especially pp. 33–51 on infant development.

Robertson J and Robertson J (1969) *Young Children in Brief Separation: John, 17 months, 9 days in a residential surgery* (Film). Tavistock Institute of Human Relations, London. (Available from Concord Film Council, Ipswich, Suffolk).

Further reading

Bateman A and Holmes J (1995) *Introduction to Psychoanalysis.* Routledge, London.

Beck AT (1976) *Cognitive Therapy and the Emotional Disorders.* International Universities Press, New York.

Berne E (1966) *Games People Play: the psychology of human relationships.* Penguin, Harmondsworth.

Burnham JB (1986) *Family Therapy: first steps towards a systemic approach.* Tavistock, London.

Caper R (1988) *Immaterial Facts: Freud's discovery of psychic reality and Klein's development of his work.* Aronson, New Jersey.

Frank J (1971) What is psychotherapy? In: S Bloch (ed) *An Introduction to the Psychotherapies.* Oxford University Press, Oxford.

Hughes P (1997) The use of countertransference in the treatment of anorexia nervosa. *European Eating Disorders Review.* **5**(4): 258–69.

Stern DN (1985) *The Interpersonal World of the Infant: a view from psychoanalysis and developmental psychology.* Basic Books, New York.

Stern R and Drummond L (1991) *The Practice of Behavioural and Cognitive Psychotherapy.* Cambridge University Press, Cambridge.

Weissman WM and Markowitz J (1994) Interpersonal psychotherapy: current status. *Archives of General Psychiatry.* **51**: 599–606.

5

Doing it: the practice of psychodynamic psychotherapy

What patients and what problems should be treated by dynamic psychotherapy? • Deciding who is likely to benefit • Patients who are less likely to benefit • Specialist resources • The setting for dynamic psychotherapy • Starting psychotherapy: negotiating the therapeutic contract • The aims of dynamic psychotherapy • The process and rules of therapy • What does the therapist do? • How long should therapy last? • Individual or group psychotherapy? • Group psychotherapy • Training in dynamic psychotherapy • The place of supervision • Evidence for the efficacy of dynamic psychotherapy • Providing a district service

What patients and what problems should be treated by dynamic psychotherapy?

MAIN POINTS

- There are a few patients who come to psychiatric or psychotherapy clinics with one symptom or one clear-cut diagnosis after a lifetime of good psychological health.

- Many patients, however, come with one or several current diagnoses in the setting of long-standing personality or interpersonal problems.

- Psychotherapy differs from general psychiatry in that the psychotherapist is less interested in a diagnostic category and more interested in the attitudes and personal characteristics which will allow the patient to benefit from therapy.

- Many patients who have NHS psychotherapy have had or are currently having psychiatric treatment, including drug treatment.

In any outpatient clinic, medical or psychiatric, you will find patients who have been well until they developed their present illness, in whom the doctor can make one clear diagnosis and for whom the recommended treatment works successfully in the expected time. This is not always the case, however.

Many patients who come to a psychiatrist have several problems and several diagnoses; some show improvement after a course of drug treatment and some have long-standing difficulties related to personality problems. Most people referred to NHS psychotherapy departments have multiple diagnoses (for example, Dolan *et al.*, 1995), and are similar to patients who attend a psychiatric outpatient clinic.

The most common presenting complaints of patients who seek psychodynamic psychotherapy are depression, anxiety and chronic or repeated relationship problems. The most common diagnostic categories of people who seek dynamic psychotherapy are:

- depressive disorder (very common)

- personality disorder/problems (very common)
- generalised anxiety state (less common)
- eating disorder (less common).

These symptoms and diagnostic categories are not necessarily indications for psychodynamic psychotherapy. Dynamic psychotherapy differs from psychiatry in that it is less interested in the diagnosis and more interested in the person's view of self and others. Thus although diagnostic categories are not ignored, the assessing psychotherapist will enquire about the patient's personality and way of relating to the world. An assessment of whether the patient will be helped by dynamic therapy will focus on attitude and capacity to use the therapy more than on categorical diagnosis or on symptoms. In many cases it is likely that the patient will also have psychiatric treatment, either at the same time or before the psychotherapy begins. This may include concurrent drug treatment. Some patients will have had previous hospital admissions.

Deciding who is likely to benefit

MAIN POINTS

- Psychodynamic psychotherapy is demanding for the patient and not everyone can benefit from the treatment.

- There are no absolutes in making a decision about whether a person can use the therapy. The assessing clinician must weigh positive and negative factors.

- Factors which are considered include the person's recognition that his problem is psychological, his motivation, sense of responsibility for himself, curiosity about himself, ability to make emotional contact, reliability and staying power.

In some aspects of medicine the patient is a relatively passive recipient of medical care. In psychodynamic psychotherapy he has to be actively engaged in the treatment for it to be effective.

The clinician assessing the patient seeking psychotherapy has to assess whether he is prepared to be actively involved in a therapy, and whether he has enough resilience in his personality (even if he is quite ill) to build on existing personality strengths and modify maladaptive attitudes. Psychodynamic psychotherapy is stressful for the patient. He has to revive memories and thoughts that he has avoided or defended against, and it is important to ensure that the patient is going to be helped and not harmed by the process.

The psychotherapist who evaluates a patient's suitability for psychotherapy is rather like an anaesthetist who assesses a patient's suitability for surgery. The patient must be ill enough to need the operation, and well enough to survive the anaesthetic. There are few absolutes in making an assessment, and the assessor will weigh several factors. The patient's preference for psychological treatment is often a consideration. In an assessment for suitability the following six points should be evaluated:

- **Recognition of a problem as psychological**. Does this person recognise that the problems have a mental or emotional component? Some people have difficulty in envisaging psychological disorder as other than a disease process.

- **Sense of responsibility for his own situation**. Does the person feel some responsibility for his life being as it is or does he see himself as a helpless victim of other people's shortcomings?

- **Curiosity or psychological mindedness**. Is this person curious about himself and does he wonder why his life has turned out as it has?

- **Motivation**. Is he motivated to work at understanding and changing his attitudes and behaviour? Note, the wish to be listened to and looked after is not the same as motivation for psychodynamic psychotherapy, which demands hard work and self-questioning from the patient.

- **Capacity to relate to another person**. Does he show some evidence of being able to make a relationship with another person, i.e. not so cut off from his own or other people's feelings that a relationship with a therapist is going to be impossible? This is clearly a matter of degree.

- **Staying power**. Is he able to turn up reasonably reliably for sessions and does he show some evidence of ability to stick at things, e.g. a job or relationship, and not to abandon it as soon as there is a problem?

Patients who are less likely to benefit

MAIN POINTS

- A person currently abusing drugs or alcohol is likely to use the substance to obliterate anxiety raised in the session.

- A person who uses impulsive acts of violence to reduce anxiety may be a danger to himself or someone else if treated in an ordinary outpatient setting.

- A person with organic brain disease cannot usually use conventional psychotherapeutic treatment.

- A person who is acutely psychotic is not usually helped by dynamic intervention in the acute phase of the illness.

- A person who has been severely deprived should be assessed with care, in case the therapy reduces rather than improves coping strategies.

- Previous overdose or self harm is *not* a contraindication for dynamic psychotherapy.

The question of who should not be offered dynamic psychotherapy involves a degree of judgement. Some people who would not be treated in an ordinary psychotherapy outpatient setting may do well in a specialist unit. Others may not benefit from therapy themselves, but their families may be helped by some sessions of family therapy or problem-based counselling to help them come to terms with a difficult situation.

The categories of patients who would not usually be helped by conventional psychodynamic psychotherapy include:

- **Someone currently abusing drugs or alcohol**. This person is dealing with anxiety by obliterating it with intoxicants. He is unlikely to use anxiety in therapy to reflect on his feelings and behaviour. Supportive group therapy may be part of a specialist rehabilitation programme. He may be suitable for psychotherapy in an ordinary outpatient setting if he can stay off addictive substances for a period of not less than 6 months.

- **Someone who habitually deals with anxiety by impulsive acts of violence**, either to himself or another person. This is different from a person who has very occasionally hit out at himself or another person. A patient who is subject to repeated acts of impulsive violence may, however, be treated in a specialist unit (see below).

- **A person with organic brain disease**, although family therapy may be useful in helping family adjustment.

- **A person with acute psychotic illness**. If a patient is introduced to dynamic psychotherapy during the acute phase of his illness, he is likely to become more disordered by having a therapy where he has to tolerate a degree of stress. A previous episode of psychosis in someone who is fully recovered is not necessarily a contra-indication, though good communication and cooperation between patient, psychiatrist and psychotherapist is essential. If a patient already in therapy suffers a psychotic breakdown the therapist and psychiatrist may judge that supportive psychotherapeutic work should continue while the patient has psychiatric treatment for his psychotic symptoms.

- **A person with a history of severe deprivation and abuse**. This is a difficult decision, because the patient may very much want psychotherapy and elicit a strong wish to respond in other people including the assessing psychotherapist. The problem in therapy is that such a person may become desperately clingy and needy when given the opportunity to become dependent. He may not be able to accept the necessary limits, including the ending, without feeling rejected and damaged. In this case a judgement must be made about how disabled this person is as a result of the deprivation, and whether a dependent therapeutic relationship will help or actually cause further harm. It is important to remember that most severely deprived people have found some way of coping with their need, and upsetting the balance by offering short-term or limited care can be unsettling, and may even reduce existing coping skills which are not then easily regained.

Note, a factor which is **not** a contraindication for psychodynamic psychotherapy is a previous suicide attempt or episodes of self-harm. Many patients who have had a history of depression or personality disorder have injured themselves. This is not in itself a reason not to offer them therapy, although the history of self-harm is important and the possible risk of a further incident should be kept in mind.

Specialist psychotherapy resources

MAIN POINTS

- Some patients who cannot be effectively treated in an ordinary NHS psychotherapy clinic may be helped with specialised treatment.

- Patients who may be helped in this way include those with learning disability and those with severe personality disorder.

- The resources to treat these patients are very limited in the NHS.

There are limited services available for people with problems that cannot normally be treated in an ordinary NHS psychotherapy clinic. People with a **mild mental handicap** can be treated by a therapist trained to work both with people with learning disability and in psychotherapy. Resources for these people are regrettably severely limited in the NHS. People with **severe personality disorders** who may not be suitable for the treatment available in a conventional clinic may be helped by having intensive treatment in a containing environment where as well as having psychotherapy, behavioural problems are repeatedly confronted within a community of mental health professionals and patients.

Patients who have severe personality disorders are often extremely expensive to the health service, to social services, to the prison services and thus to the community as a whole. There is in addition an intergenerational impact on their children who suffer the short- and long-term effects of their parents' disturbed behaviour. Treatments in these specialised settings have been shown to be cost effective (Menzies *et al.*, 1993). However, because the cost of treatment is taken from local health budgets, and the cost of other interventions from social services and prison budgets, it may be cheaper for the local health authority to withhold treatment and allow other services to take over. As a result, some of these important resources are intermittently threatened with closure.

The setting for dynamic psychotherapy

MAIN POINTS

- A reliable and predictable setting allows the patient to feel secure to explore new ideas.
- The setting should be comfortable, quiet and uninterrupted.

The setting for psychotherapy should be reliable, predictable, quiet and uninterrupted. There are two particular reasons for taking some care with the setting for psychotherapy:

1 the patient is more likely to feel able to explore new ideas if he feels secure, and is in a predictable environment

2 the predictability and invariability of the setting highlights any changes which the patient himself tries to make, and gives clues to his inner world.

It may seem obvious that the patient should see the *same therapist* for each session, but this is not the norm in many other medical settings. The relationship between the therapist and patient is different from other medical or nursing relationships. Because the therapeutic relationship is so important to the therapy, the therapist has to be there for treatment to take place. This means, for example, that the therapist cannot go on holiday or take a day away at a conference and expect someone else to cover. Instead the therapy session must either be cancelled or the time rearranged.

The *time* of the therapy is usually arranged, as far as possible, to be the same from week to week. There may occasionally need to be some flexibility to accommodate other commitments for either patient or therapist, but the patient's request for changed times or his feelings about the therapist's request for a change should be discussed and analysed in the therapy.

The *place* where therapy takes place should be the same for each session. It should be reasonably *quiet* and at the very least the conversation in the room should not be audible outside. The sessions should *not be interrupted*, which may mean arranging for phone calls to be diverted until after the session, and if the therapist carries a bleeper she should arrange to have it covered by another person for the time of the session.

Starting psychotherapy: negotiating the therapeutic contract

MAIN POINTS

- A person beginning dynamic psychotherapy should have an explanation of what to expect from the therapy.

- The therapist should clarify the broad aims of the therapy, the rules and process the patient should anticipate, and what the patient hopes and expects to achieve from the treatment.

Many people are anxious when they arrive for a first psychotherapy appointment, unsure of what to expect. In the preliminary session before starting the therapy proper the therapist should discuss and explore some important areas with the patient. The patient's active involvement is essential for therapy, and he needs to know what can be achieved, what he can expect from the therapist and what he himself will be expected to contribute.

At the beginning of therapy the therapist should:

- explore what the patient wants from the treatment and discuss the overall aims of this kind of therapy

- explain what happens in therapy and what the rules of the relationship are

- clarify what the patient himself can realistically expect from the treatment and negotiate a therapeutic contract (working alliance).

The aims of dynamic psychotherapy

MAIN POINTS

The overall aims of dynamic psychotherapy are:

- to increase the person's awareness of his patterns of behaviour

- to help the person be aware of and take responsibility for what he contributes to his difficulties

- to help the person be more aware of his conscious and unconscious expectations and his motives in maintaining damaging patterns of behaviour

- to help the person have more control and more choice in his life

- to help the person have better self-esteem.

The therapy should help the patient see what patterns of behaviour are repeated in his life and what he himself is contributing to his difficulties. If the patient can get a better understanding of the background to his problems and of his conscious and unconscious motives in maintaining maladaptive solutions, he will have more choice about alternative ways of behaving, thinking and feeling.

Psychodynamic therapy does not seek to apportion blame, either to the patient or to his family. It does aim to help the patient to see where responsibility lies, and to take responsibility for himself as he now is, so that he can be more effective in directing his life.

Commonly people who have been troubled by long-standing or even recent psychological problems feel ashamed, guilty or inadequate about their situation. The therapist's willingness to be interested and to spend time listening and helping make sense of the issues is useful in itself. The experience of being taken seriously and listened to thoughtfully is an important factor in restoring self-esteem and self-confidence.

The process and rules of therapy

MAIN POINTS

- The therapy is a serious commitment for both patient and therapist.

- There should be an agreement, if appropriate, about the duration of therapy.

- The therapist will not behave as in a social relationship.

- The patient may want to discuss whether it is acceptable to get psychotropic medication from the GP or psychiatrist while in therapy.

Commitment

This is a serious commitment for both patient and therapist. The therapist will tell the patient that sessions will begin and end on time and that he will not cancel a session if it can be avoided. He will give as much warning as possible about holidays or other breaks. The patient is asked to show the same reliability about being on time and not cancelling a session lightly. The patient should be given a contact telephone number to let the therapist know if he is unable to keep an appointment or will be delayed. The therapist should have a contact number for the patient for the same reason.

Length of therapy

The time and place and the length of therapy have to be agreed at the beginning of the therapy. In the NHS, the patient does not usually have much control over how long the therapy lasts. Limited resources usually means that therapy has a time limit from the outset. In the private sector the length of therapy may be negotiated, and patient and therapist together are likely to decide when the therapy should come to an end.

How the patient should expect the therapist to behave

The patient should be told at the beginning of therapy that this is different from a social relationship. The focus will be on what is on his mind, and on what he is feeling and thinking, and he should be warned that the therapist will expect to keep the focus on his feelings and thoughts and may not respond, for example, to social questions.

Negotiating a contract: the working alliance

An important first step is to establish a realistic contract with the patient (working alliance) where the work of treatment is recognised as a partnership in which therapist and patient work together against the problems.

Three issues should be addressed:

1 that the patient can come regularly to sessions

2 that his expectations are realistic

3 that he is responsible for doing a lot of the work of therapy.

At the minimum the patient has to agree that he can come regularly to sessions, and that he can talk about his thoughts and feelings. In addition, however, it is useful to address two common misconceptions which people starting therapy may have. First, that there will be rapid relief from long-standing problems, and second, that the change will come from the therapist or the environment rather than from within the patient himself.

It is also useful to get some idea of what the patient's hopes are for the effect of the therapy. It may be clear that the patient is unrealistic in expecting more than can be achieved in the time and with the treatment available, and this should be discussed early if it is not to be a risk factor in the therapy breaking down.

Of course, discussion does not necessarily resolve such misconceptions, but it puts them on the agenda for further examination, and establishes that the therapist will not collude in an idealisation of therapy, and will not be a helpless victim when the idealisation inevitably collapses.

Concurrent treatment

Some people who seek psychotherapy are also being treated by a GP or psychiatrist for psychiatric symptoms and may be taking prescribed drugs. If a patient is suffering distressing symptoms it is hard to argue that they should not receive any treatment which is likely to alleviate the symptoms, and most psychotherapists support the concurrent use of drug treatment and psychotherapy, provided this combined treatment is in the patient's interest. It is important in this situation that good communication between psychotherapist and GP or psychiatrist is maintained. The patient should not be left feeling that he is being disloyal to the one by attending the other.

There are two situations in which a psychotherapist may suggest that it is not in the patient's interest to take prescribed drugs while having psychotherapy.

1 If the patient is on so much psychoactive medication that his thinking is impaired or his affective responses seriously blunted, then he will be less accessible for reflection about his state of mind during therapy. In this case the benefits of the drug must be balanced against the benefits of the therapy.

2 If the patient does not seem to get great symptomatic benefit from the drug, but is manifestly using it as 'comfort' and as something to depend on which will always be available. This sometimes happens when the patient is reluctant to look at issues around dependency in therapy and uses the drug to obliterate anxiety aroused by feeling a sense of need for another person.

What does the therapist do?

MAIN POINTS

- The therapist is active in the sessions both in her attentiveness and in her interventions and communications to the patient.

- The demands of the therapeutic relationship mean that the therapist should be emotionally available but not be prepared to engage in a social relationship with the patient either outside or inside the therapeutic time.

- The therapist is constantly reflective about her emotional response to the patient and on what this says about the patient's conscious and unconscious expectations and assumptions. The therapist refrains from acting on the feelings aroused but rather uses these feelings and thoughts to communicate a greater self-understanding to the patient.

The therapist does three things throughout the therapy:

1 *interacts* with the patient in ways which will help him to achieve the aims of the therapy, that is to become more reflective and more aware of his own behaviours, feelings and motives. The therapist is attentive and makes interventions

2 *maintains* the boundaries of the therapy

3 *maintains in herself a state of mind* which is both receptive and reflective.

Interacting with the patient

The idea of the therapist as a silent spectator or passive recipient of the patient's projections is a caricature of the therapeutic process. The therapist is neither silent nor passive but actively:

- *listens* to what is said
- *notices* behaviour and non-verbal cues
- *observes* the atmosphere of the session and the feelings which the patient evokes in the therapist from moment to moment
- *responds* to the patient's various communications.

Interventions

The overall aim of the therapy is to help the patient understand himself better and to change his internal (mental) representations of self and others, and the therapist uses a variety of interventions. The therapist may:

- ask the patient to *clarify* facts
- *encourage* the patient to explore an important issue, that is to be more reflective

- *confront* the patient with an important aspect or consequence of his behaviour which is being consciously evaded or unconsciously avoided

- *interpret* behaviour or feelings by offering an alternative way of thinking about it, which may include suggesting that the patient's behaviour is influenced by thoughts or feelings which are not fully conscious

- *empathise* with a patient's feelings so that the patient knows that his state of mind is recognised

- at times and particularly with some self-destructive patients, the therapist may decide to offer active *approval* of constructive change which the patient has made

- *giving advice* is not part of a psychoanalytic approach, but occasionally a patient will be helped by a suggestion from the therapist about a decision or action to be taken.

Clinical example

The patient, Paul, is a 26-year-old man who has suffered disabling spells of depression and has not been able to achieve his potential at work. His social life is limited and he lives with his elderly parents, who worry about him and are openly critical of his failure to deal with his problems.

This is the sixth session. He has been explaining how irritated he feels with the neighbours who look down on him and his family, but who are a worthless lot living on income support.

Patient: They're really rude to me, not you know, openly, but the way they talk to me, and sometimes ignore the fact that I'm in the room.

Therapist: When did that happen?

Patient: About a month ago. Mrs W came over, just popped in. I was watching the television and she didn't even say hello to me, just sat down and began to talk to my Mum.

Therapist: And what did you do?

Patient: I sat there. And felt angry. She was so rude, and they think they're better than me just because their son went to university. I didn't say anything, but I felt angry all right. And after a bit I went up to my room and lay on the bed till she went. Then my Mum came up and complained that I had been rude to Mrs W. So we had a row.

The patient has made a rather general complaint about neighbours he disliked, and the therapist asks him to *explain*, and to be specific about an occasion when he felt badly treated. This asks him to give a much fuller and more specific description of his feelings and behaviours.

Therapist: So then you felt criticised by your mother as well as by Mrs W.
Patient: Yes.
Therapist: That must have been difficult.

Here the therapist empathises with the patient's distress. She has chosen not to address several issues in the story.

Therapist: It seems from what you have told me today and other days that you often feel that people look down on you because you do not have academic qualifications. I wonder if you yourself feel quite bad about not doing better at school.
Patient: I know I should have done. I read a lot, and I know there's a lot there, in my head.

She *interprets* that the main criticism comes from within himself. Earlier the therapist could have shared the mother's irritation with her son's passive aggression. She chose, however, to make an *empathic* response to the patient's distress rather than responding to his aggression. This increased his trust of her and allowed him to respond to her identifying a difficult area, his humiliating failure at school.

Maintaining the boundaries

There are two aspects to maintaining boundaries: avoiding social involvement and protecting the therapy from external intrusions.

The therapist should ensure that a clear distinction is drawn between the 'as if' world of the therapy and the real world outside. Therapy is a time for the patient to explore and experiment with thoughts and feelings in a safe environment, and if the patient is allowed to see the relationship as a potentially social one this freedom is lost. The therapist can attend to the boundaries of therapy by paying close attention to the structure of the sessions with the patient, and ensuring their reliability in time and place. She should protect the professional therapeutic relationship and should not for example accept invitations to meet outside, nor accept gifts from the patient during the therapy.

A further aspect of boundary maintenance lies in protecting the therapeutic 'space' from intrusions. This may be simply noise or telephone calls but may also involve anxious or curious contact from relatives of the patient. These can be dealt with courteously but without disclosing any private information. It is usually appropriate to let the patient know that a family member has been in touch, so that the patient is aware of any contact that the therapist has had with his outside life.

Paul, the young man in the story above, had been in weekly psychotherapy with the active encouragement of his parents. After about eight weeks of therapy his father phoned the therapist to ask how his son was getting on. The therapist was sympathetic about his worry but explained that she could not discuss the patient or his therapy with his father. She also said that she would mention to the patient that his father had been concerned and had phoned about him. The father was dismayed and had thought that he could enter into a secret 'parental' alliance with the therapist. Discussion with the patient led to an exploration of his ambivalent wish to be dependent but also to separate from his parents.

Maintaining a reflective state of mind

Our mental representations of ourselves and others give us a map which organises our expectations. These representations can be thought of as internal dramas through which we have established habitual ways of relating to the world. We repeat certain patterns even when they are clearly maladaptive or self-destructive, e.g.

repeatedly becoming 'accidentally' pregnant, repeatedly choosing an emotionally abusive partner, repeatedly failing important exams.

In psychodynamic therapy the therapist wants to identify the conscious and unconscious beliefs which maintain these repetitive ways of behaving. We are all skilled, usually unconsciously, at finding partners in our social dramas (the sympathetic but ineffective friend, the unkind spouse, the doormat wife) and there is a danger with any new relationship that it will repeat a familiar partnership where nothing changes. The therapist breaks this cycle and establishes a relationship which allows the patient to try new ways of relating by not responding in the usual and expected manner. This is not always easy and requires that the therapist relinquishes her own wish to respond spontaneously.

The therapist should be pleasant, attentive, and focused on the patient and on what he does and what he says, but should abstain from ordinary social chat. She must be in touch with what she herself is feeling, constantly reflect on the patient's state of mind, and be careful about how she responds with her own feelings and thoughts. The main purpose of her communications to the patient is to increase the patient's self-understanding.

The therapist does not remain silent, refuse to answer all questions or always decline to offer an opinion. The relationship is a human one, but it is important that the therapist neither burdens the patient with her own problems, nor gives so much personal information that she blocks the patient's opportunity to project his own mental images on to the external person of the therapist.

Let us return to Paul, the patient in the previous vignette.

Paul arrived 10 minutes late for his seventh session, out of breath and visibly anxious. He apologised profusely and explained that it had not been his fault because his father had given him a lift and there had been a 20-minute traffic hold-up on the main road. The therapist asked where the traffic jam had been and discovered that it was about 300 yards from the outpatient department. Her immediate internal response was irritation that Paul had sat stuck in traffic for 20 minutes while he could have walked the distance in five. On reflection, however, she wondered what he was communicating. He had elicited irritation as he did with his parents. One of his presenting complaints had been that he was stuck in his life and not getting where he should be, and could not understand what he could do about it. She decided she should acknowledge his expectation that she would be angry about the lateness and point out his ability to unwittingly sabotage his own attempts to get treatment. She thought that at this stage in the therapy Paul would not be able to take in any interpretation about the possible hostility implicit in the avoidable lateness, but that he might be able to think about his own agency in being stuck.

Therapist: You seem to expect me to tell you off for lateness.
Patient: Yes, yes I do, I'm sorry, I didn't set out to be late.
Therapist: And even though you can see now that I'm not upset or angry but curious about your lateness you're still anxious.
Patient: I'm sorry, I didn't mean it, I left in good time.
Therapist: The thing that I'm interested in is why you had to stay stuck in the car with your father when you could have got out. It looks as though you have no confidence that you can take action to sort anything out.

The therapist was conscious of her irritation but rather than retaliating and criticising the patient for wasting her time, or for incompetence, she let him know that she was aware that he expected her to feel attacked by his lateness, but that she did not feel hurt and was not going to retaliate. She was, however, confronting *about the consequences of his passivity, although indicating that her interest was in understanding why he could not solve his problems with getting stuck. She also alluded to his staying with his father, with the intention of returning to this point later, suspecting that separation from his parents was an issue for him.*

How long should therapy last?

MAIN POINTS

- Short-term therapy for up to 20 sessions is indicated for patients with adequate previous adjustment and focused symptoms.

continued ...

- Patients with long-standing and more severe symptoms or inter-personal problems need longer-term therapy of 40 sessions or more.

- Patients with severe and long-standing personality disorder bene-fit from intensive specialist day hospital or inpatient treatment, with the programme of treatment lasting at least two years.

- In a publicly funded health service limited resources may restrict what can be offered to a patient.

- Psychoanalysis is the most intense and demanding form of dynamic psychotherapy. It is not available in the NHS.

Short-term psychotherapy

This is usually defined as up to 20 sessions. A brief intervention is suitable for the patient who has had previously adequate psycho-logical health and adjustment, and who has a specific symptom or problem with a definable onset. The therapy will usually focus on a specific problem.

In addition, some patients who have more extensive interpersonal problems do not want more than a limited number of sessions, and good work can be done in this time, as long as the patient and therapist are realistic about what can be achieved.

Long-term psychotherapy

When the patient has long-standing psychological difficulties, especially when there is evidence that there are moderate to severe personality problems, then longer-term therapy at least once a week for one year or more is indicated.

Patients with the most severe personality disorders may need concurrent support from psychiatric services and may benefit from intensive psychodynamic treatment in a specialist day hospital or inpatient unit.

Psychoanalysis

Psychoanalysis is more ambitious than other forms of dynamic psychotherapy and aims at a more extensive restructuring of the personality. The patient has sessions four or five times a week for at least two years and sometimes for much longer. This therapy is demanding for the patient who will experience an intense and at times regressed dependent relationship with the analyst, but at the same time the frequent sessions also give support and encouragement.

Psychoanalysis is not usually available in the UK in the NHS but a number of psychoanalytic or related organisations offer subsidised treatment to patients who are likely to benefit from this approach.

Individual or group psychotherapy?

MAIN POINTS

- Many patients will benefit from either individual or group therapy.

- The real social aspects of group therapy allow direct feedback and practising interpersonal relating.

- Some narcissistic people cannot tolerate either feedback or sharing in groups.

- Some intensely socially anxious people cannot tolerate groups.

- Some people have a particular problem with intimate relationships which may be best addressed in individual therapy.

Psychodynamic therapy may be offered in an individual or group setting. Many patients will benefit from either. Some have a strong preference for one or other.

Advantages of group therapy

- The social setting of group therapy invites the person to behave in the usual way.

- There is a reality about issues like sharing which have to be resolved and bring up important concerns for most people.

- The group will offer many opportunities for different interaction.

- The person realises that his problem is not unique.

- There is often overt support between group members which is not possible or appropriate in individual therapy.

- There is direct feedback about behaviour from other group members.

- One group member may bring up an issue which is difficult for another person and facilitate exploration.

- In a group a person may see his own behaviour mirrored when someone else does it.

Possible difficulties in group therapy

- Some narcissistic or very anxious people cannot tolerate exposure.

- There is less opportunity to explore problems of being closely involved with one person than there is in individual therapy.

- Some people have difficulty in taking time for themselves in competition with others.

- Conversely some have great difficulty in allowing anyone else to have time.

Some of these problems can be resolved in the group, which may indeed be an ideal place to do this, but while most people enjoy group therapy once they have overcome their initial anxiety, there are others whose continuing anxiety or anger will block progress, and who need the relative quiet of individual treatment. There are also people whose predominant problem is related to intimacy with another person for whom individual therapy is the best approach.

Advantages of individual therapy

- The person can decide his own agenda.

- There is opportunity to develop a strong therapeutic relationship with the therapist, and this is a focus for analysing wishes and fears in intimate relationships.

- For those patients who will certainly invite rejection it may be necessary to protect them with a therapist who will tolerate behaviour which would not be tolerable in a group. It may also be important that the patient can test limits in a safer setting than a group can provide.

Group psychotherapy

MAIN POINTS

- Group therapy is practised by therapists with different theoretical backgrounds.

- Most group psychotherapy currently available in the UK uses a psychodynamic approach.

- Group therapy works by giving people the opportunity to enact their habitual relationships in a safe 'social' setting where the interaction can be analysed and understood.

- Therapy groups may be homogeneous, including only patients with a shared problem, or may be heterogeneous, including people with a range of different problems.

- Common anxieties for people starting group therapy include fear of rejection, of being made worse and of being ridiculed.

Group psychotherapy is not, strictly speaking, part of the classificatory system, because by definition it relates more to structure than to a consistent technique. The broad category of 'group psychotherapy' includes, however, group analysis, which derives directly from psychoanalytic principles. Group analysis was initially proposed and practised by the psychoanalyst Michael Foulkes. His ideas on the possible therapeutic effects of group treatments followed from his work with servicemen wounded in the Second World War. A similar psychoanalytic approach to group psychotherapy, which also developed from work with wounded servicemen in the Second World War, was practised by Wilfred Bion.

Group psychotherapy seeks to include not only an exploration of the individual's mental representations, but also has an interest in social interaction and demonstration of interpersonal problems in a social setting. Group psychotherapy thus also has something in common with systemic therapy.

We are brought up in social and family groups and the expectations and assumptions we bring to relationships outside the family, in school, at work and in our friendships will have been crucially influenced by our earlier experiences of socialisation. Most group therapy at present available in the UK is based on a dynamic tradition but is also practised by therapists trained in cognitive therapy.

Psychodynamic group therapy incorporates many of the principles of individual psychodynamic psychotherapy. The aims of the therapy are to help the patient understand more about his conscious and unconscious feelings and to improve his self-esteem. Patients are generally selected in the same way as for individual therapy and using the same criteria, and the same careful attention is paid to the setting.

How does psychodynamic group therapy work?

- Family relationships are inevitably repeated in a group, but there is the opportunity to think about what is happening and to try to understand the assumptions that each person brings to the various relationships in the group. Why is A attracted to B while finding C so irritating? Why does D so anxiously try to sit inconspicuously? Why is B often maternal and protective to D?

- For many people, the experience of finding that other people can suffer anxiety, uncertainty or other problems can be reassuring. Often people have a sense of being very isolated in their lives, imagining that others manage personal difficulties easily and that they are to blame for not managing better. Realising that life problems are universal is sometimes useful in helping people to stop blaming themselves and have the confidence to work out solutions.

Structure and process of therapy groups

- There are usually 6–10 group members.
- There are one or two group conductors or leaders.
- The group meets once or twice a week for 1–1½ hours.
- The duration of the therapy is from a few weeks to several years.
- A group may be open or closed. A closed group runs with a fixed membership which will not change; an open group will replace members who leave. The most usual format is the slow-open group in which a member will leave infrequently, say one to three a year, and each will be replaced by a new member.

Different kinds of group

- Outpatient psychotherapy groups of people who have sought therapy for various interpersonal problems (see above, under 'Which patients?').
- Supportive groups for people with a shared problem, e.g. Alcoholics Anonymous, CRUSE groups for the bereaved, etc.

Common anxieties about groups

- Fear of rejection.
- Fear of being made more sick by meeting other 'problem' people.
- Fear of exposure and ridicule.

These anxieties are universal and should be explored with the patient in the preliminary interview.

Training in dynamic psychotherapy

MAIN POINTS

- Psychotherapy is an umbrella term for psychological treatment that includes the listening skills which any nurse or doctor should have.

- Formal training in psychotherapy in the UK is now regulated by two bodies, the United Kingdom Council for Psychotherapy and the British Confederation of Psychotherapists.

- Training in psychotherapy includes personal therapy, academic learning and supervised clinical practice.

- Psychotherapy is psychologically demanding work with pitfalls for the poorly trained. Certain personal qualities are important for those intending to train.

The term 'psychotherapy' is sometimes used as a kind of umbrella term for psychological treatment, in which case we can assume that a good deal of psychotherapy in its broadest sense is done by nurses, doctors and others in primary care, and by psychiatrists, mental health nurses and other health professionals as well as those who have undergone a formal psychotherapy training.

Cawley in 1977 provided helpful classification in outlining three levels of 'psychotherapy' which he thought operated in medical practice, and which he classified on the professional background and training of the practitioner.

Level 1

Level 1 is what any good nurse, doctor or other health care professional does and is an important part of the art of medicine. It involves:

- an awareness of the person as well as the problem
- an ability to communicate and empathise with people from different backgrounds
- an ability to recognise the patient's anxieties
- the ability to help the patient with anxiety by explaining the problem and reducing irrational fear.

Level 2

Level 2 is what a person trained in psychiatric care (for example, psychiatrist, psychiatric nurse, clinical psychologist) does. Counselling would be a sophisticated version of this level. It includes everything in Level 1 but also requires:

- an ability to understand and communicate with patients suffering from all kinds of psychological disturbance
- a recognition that the person's present state of mind is influenced by previous experience, often in ways of which he is unaware
- an awareness of the phenomenon of transference which will not, however, be used in the therapy except in the sense of allowing a mildly positive transference (seeing the doctor as a good and reliable 'parent') to reinforce the therapeutic relationship (see p. 79 for discussion of what is meant by 'transference').

Level 3

Level 3 would be what most people mean by psychodynamic psychotherapy in its formal sense. It includes the characteristics of levels 1 and 2 which relate to the therapist's attitude to the patient, i.e. respect, understanding and acceptance. It also includes:

- helping the patient to face the truth about himself and his responsibility for himself and his relationships

- focusing on the therapist–patient relationship in order to explore and understand the patient's problems

- encouraging the development of transference and actively working with it in order to elucidate unconscious feelings which affect the person's present.

We can see from this list that training in psychotherapy at its broadest includes training in communication skills which is now expected for undergraduate medical and nursing students. Much of this is at the level of social skills training and ideally should include addressing the problem of how a difficult patient or a difficult situation can make a professional become anxious and perhaps defensive and clumsy.

Postgraduate trainees in psychiatry in the UK are required to have supervised experience of seeing patients for psychotherapy, both behavioural and psychodynamic. The theory of psychodynamic psychotherapy forms part of the curriculum for the membership exam of the Royal College of Psychiatrists. At present there is no such requirement for postgraduate nursing training, although many psychiatric nurses choose to have some further training in psychotherapy.

Recognition of training in psychotherapy

Until 1993 there was no regulatory body in the UK to monitor the practice of psychotherapy. There are now two bodies which register training organisations. These are the United Kingdom Council for Psychotherapy (UKCP) and the British Confederation of Psychotherapists (BCP).

Formal training in psychodynamic psychotherapy

All reputable training organisations have three parts to their training. These include:

- personal therapy from a therapist recognised by the training organisation
- theoretical learning usually in the form of reading seminars
- supervised clinical practice, with a supervisor or supervisors recognised by the training organisation.

Training organisations differ in their requirements for personal therapy and clinical experience. The most intensive trainings, for example at the Institute of Psycho-Analysis, require the trainee to be in personal analysis five times a week for at least three years, and to have two patients in five-times-a-week analysis for one and two years. Other training organisations require personal therapy or analysis between one and four times a week, usually for not less than three years. The requirement for clinical experience is usually in line with the regulations for personal therapy.

All trainings look good on paper. The quality of the training is influenced by the rigour of its selection of candidates, and the quality of the therapy and supervision. It will be immediately obvious that these are related. Inevitably those organisations which take all applicants or which require only an academic qualification end up with a certain number of unsuitable trainees and eventually unsuitable therapists.

Qualities needed to work as a psychotherapist

- A minimum academic qualification, usually university degree or equivalent professional training.
- Ability to empathise with other people's states of mind.
- Ability to communicate this empathy to another person without being sentimental.

- Ability to remain calm and continue to think rationally when confronted by another person's disturbed thinking.

- Ability to avoid being drawn into enactments of a patient's wishes, especially when these involve a violation of the therapeutic boundary.

- Ability to reflect on one's own feelings without feeling compelled to act on these.

- A sufficiently rewarding personal life which will both support the therapist and allow a capacity to maintain a healthy distance from the patients. The therapist should not *need* his or her patients.

This is a personal list drawn up by the author, who is not aware of any such published guidelines in a training organisation.

The place of supervision

MAIN POINTS

- A therapist will get many projections of painful feelings from her patients, particularly in a psychiatric setting where she may be working with very disturbed patients.

- One way to help an inexperienced therapist recognise what is being unconsciously enacted in the relationship with the patient is by having supervision from an experienced psychotherapist.

- Supervision is an important aspect of training for junior doctors and nurses in psychiatry.

Psychodynamic psychotherapy uses the therapeutic relationship to allow the patient to express aspects of his inner representational world by projecting aspects of this on to the person of the therapist. The therapist in turn is alert to the feelings aroused in her by the patient and his communications.

An obvious potential pitfall in this relationship is that the therapist has an inner world and her own propensity to recreate internal relationships. Having personal therapy is one way to find out more about our unconscious needs and wishes, to be able to recognise at least some of our own assumptions and expectations, and thus to have more control over them.

Personal therapy is a requirement for professional psychotherapists, but not for other professionals who work with psychologically disturbed people and who offer patients limited psychotherapy (see above). It is not feasible for all psychiatric nurses or junior doctors to have personal therapy or analysis and some professionals may not wish to have therapy. It is therefore very helpful for an inexperienced therapist, and important for the therapeutic outcome, that the therapist has supervision of her work from an experienced practitioner.

In an NHS setting, supervision is usually weekly, with four or five trainees working together in a group with a supervisor. Therapists write a detailed account of the sessions, describing what the patient said, what the therapist said, and the feelings expressed by the patient and aroused in the therapist. This clinical account is discussed by the group, with the supervisor helping the therapist to identify the patient's projections and to understand what is being communicated.

Outside the formal psychotherapeutic setting many disturbed patients project painful affect into the staff who work with them, often leaving staff not only depressed or angry but even confused. Any staff who work with disturbed patients should have some opportunity to learn to disentangle their own feelings and thoughts from those which are elicited by the patient, and which largely belong to the patient's model of the world.

Example: *A young woman with a history of repeated self-injury and a long-standing eating disorder was a patient in a day hospital. When she heard that her key worker, a staff nurse on the unit, was leaving in a few weeks time to move to another hospital, she became abusive and denigrating, telling the nurse angrily that the treatment had been useless and that the nurse should be reported for malpractice. The nurse initially felt hurt and depressed by her inability to help the patient. On reflection she realised that the patient was projecting her own sense of rejection and depression into her. With the realisation that the distress truly belonged to the patient she felt her self-esteem less diminished, and was able to make contact with the patient and to acknowledge the patient's feelings of hurt and disappointment.*

Training in thinking about one's personal response to a patient is an essential part of psychotherapy supervision. It is a valuable learning experience for the junior doctor or nurse who gradually acquires the ability to recognise some of the subliminal communications of a patient, and who also becomes more alert to her own cognitive and affective responses.

Evidence for the efficacy of dynamic psychotherapy

MAIN POINTS

- Efficacy and effectiveness are not the same.

- There are methodological problems in psychotherapy research which are related to difficulties in standardising both the patient characteristics and the therapeutic intervention.

- There is lot of research on the efficacy of psychotherapy in general and a smaller amount demonstrating the efficacy of dynamic psychotherapy.

There is a distinction between the efficacy and the effectiveness of any treatment.

- *Efficacy* is the effect of the intervention in a research setting.

- *Effectiveness* is the outcome of the intervention in real clinical practice.

This is an important distinction because as all clinicians know, the patients who seek treatment in the GP's surgery or the outpatient clinic are often different from the 'standard' patient of the published trial.

Methodological issues in assessing the outcome of psychotherapy research

- **Comorbidity**: Patients who are selected for a trial of a treatment intervention may not be representative of all patients with the same problem. In real life, patients have an inconvenient habit of having several problems at the same time. Studies of patients who attend for psychotherapy have shown that there is a high level of co-morbidity (for example, Dolan *et al.*, 1995). That is, using ICD 10 or DSM IV criteria, the patients have symptoms which put them into several diagnostic categories at once. Thus an intervention which has been shown to be effective in depression, for example, may not be entirely satisfactory in a patient who has symptoms of depression, eating disorder and personality disorder at the same time.

- **Patient preference and motivation**: If the patient is part of a randomised controlled trial, he does not usually have a choice about which therapy he will receive. In a clinical setting the patient's preference for any approach will be a strong factor in deciding which treatment he will have. This motivation is likely to affect outcome and will compromise trial results.

- **Therapist difference**: While standardisation of intervention is relatively straightforward for drug trials, there is a particular problem with a treatment where the intervention includes a human relationship as an important part of the treatment. Variables include quality of the therapist's training, length of experience, skill of the therapist, and 'fit' between therapist and patient.

- **Outcome measures**: Some psychotherapists are reluctant to use conventional measures of mental disorder, such as psychometric scales, because they offer only a crude evaluation of the complexity of the patient's inner world. Although this is a valid argument, the pressure to produce evidence of change has led to an increasing acceptance among psychotherapy researchers of the need to use symptom checklists, and to the development of more sophisticated systematic assessments (Luborsky *et al.*, 1988).

Despite these problems, there is a large body of research on the efficacy of psychotherapy in general and a smaller amount on the efficacy of dynamic psychotherapy. For example, Gabbard *et al.* (1997) reviewed the impact of providing psychotherapy for psychiatric disorders on costs of care. They examined 18 studies where there was a comparison group and where there were measures of cost in the outcome data. They found that in 80% of the 10 clinical trials with random assignment and 100% of eight trials with non-random assignment psychotherapy reduced total costs.

Crits-Cristoph (1992) reviewed 11 well-conducted studies of brief dynamic psychotherapy of 12 or more sessions which included a control group, used therapists trained in brief dynamic therapy and which gave enough information to calculate effect size. Outcome measures were target symptoms, psychiatric symptoms and social functioning. Brief dynamic psychotherapy demonstrated large effects relative to waiting-list groups, slight superiority to non-psychiatric treatments and effects about equal to other psychotherapies and medication.

Thompson *et al.* (1987) showed that brief dynamic therapy was as effective as behaviour therapies in the treatment of depression in older people. Shapiro *et al.* (1994) found that dynamic therapy was as effective as cognitive therapy in the treatment of depressed outpatients.

It is important that research into dynamic therapy continues. Future research should focus on discovering more precisely which symptoms and patterns of behaviour respond best to which kind of psychotherapy, and what the optimal number of sessions is for effective treatment.

For a full discussion of the subject read *What Works for Whom?* (Roth and Fonagy, 1996) and *Who Will Benefit From Psychotherapy? Predicting therapeutic outcomes* (Luborsky *et al.*, 1988).

Providing a district service

MAIN POINTS

- A district service should recognise both the needs of patients and the educational needs of staff.

- Ideally, a range of therapies should be available for the local population.

- Supervised experience and academic teaching should be available for mental health professionals.

- Staff working in community or specialist teams appreciate regular discussion of clinical problems and supervision of ongoing work.

- Contact with general practice should include ease of access for the GPs and opportunities for two-way education.

A psychotherapy service needs to address the needs of both patients and staff. Staff should have regular opportunity for discussion of difficult cases, clinical supervision for those who seek further experience and good liaison with community mental health teams so that referral of a patient in either direction is straightforward. Some staff will be required to have supervised clinical experience (Royal College of Psychiatrists' regulations for trainees in psychiatry) and others will ask for such experience as part of their postgraduate training.

Contact with GPs is logistically more difficult. At the least, the GP should get regular information about how to contact the service and how to refer a patient. Psychotherapists and GPs can learn from each other and there is scope for educational meetings for shared teaching.

Ideally, a psychotherapy service in the NHS should include the following:

- training of all doctors, nurses and other mental health workers to a level where they can offer psychodynamically informed treatment to all their patients and psychodynamically informed support to their junior staff

- a readily available counselling service within the community to deal with immediate problems and to help make decisions about future referral

- short-term therapies including cognitive, behavioural, brief dynamic and interpersonal therapies for those patients who have an identifiable specific problem

- longer-term cognitive and dynamic therapy, both individual and group, for those who have more extensive interpersonal problems, but who have generally had a fair level of psychosocial functioning

- intensive longer-term treatment for those with long-standing intractable personality problems

- family therapy where family issues are clearly a part of the pathology

- regular liaison meetings between a specialist psychotherapist and mental health teams for case discussion, supervision and support

- consultation service to related organisations like general practices and social services, who share the caseload and many of the problems of the NHS.

References

Cawley RH (1977) The teaching of psychotherapy. *Association of Teachers of Psychiatry Newsletter*. 19–36.

Crits-Cristoph P (1992) The efficacy of brief dynamic psychotherapy: a meta-analysis. *American Journal of Psychiatry*. **149**(2): 151–8.

Dolan B, Evans C and Norton K (1995) Multiple axis-II diagnoses of personality disorder. *British Journal of Psychiatry*. **166**: 107–12.

Gabbard GO, Lazar SG, Hornberger J and Spiegel D (1997) The economic impact of psychotherapy: a review. *American Journal of Psychotherapy*. **154**(2): 147–55.

Luborsky L, Crits-Cristoph P, Mintz J and Auerbach A (1988) *Who Will Benefit From Psychotherapy? Predicting therapeutic outcomes.* Basic Books, New York.

Menzies D, Dolan B and Norton K (1993) Are short-term savings worth long-term costs? Funding treatment for personality disorders. *Psychiatric Bulletin.* **17**: 517–19.

Roth A and Fonagy P (1996) *What Works for Whom? A critical review of psychotherapy research.* Guilford Press, New York.

Thompson LW, Gallagher D and Breckenridge JS (1987) Comparative effectiveness of psychotherapies for depressed elders. *Journal of Consulting and Clinical Psychology.* **55**: 385–90.

Further reading

Bateman A (1997) *Outcome of a day hospital programme in the treatment of borderline personality disorder: a controlled study.* Paper presented at the Royal College of Psychiatrists Winter Meeting, 1997. Submitted for publication.

Pines M (ed) (1983) *The Evolution of Group Analysis.* Routledge and Kegan Paul, London.

Shapiro DA, Barkham M, Rees A *et al.* (1994) Effects of treatment duration and severity of depression on the effectiveness of cognitive-behavioural and psychodynamic interpersonal psychotherapy. *Journal of Consulting and Clinical Psychology.* **62**: 522–34.

6

Conclusion

Like medicine and nursing, skill in psychotherapy only comes with a long commitment to study and practice. Neither acquiring the skill nor having the treatment is an easy option. Some people seek psychological treatment hoping that there is a magical cure for their long-standing mental or emotional problems. Magical treatments are certainly on the market and enjoy some popularity. The mainstream psychological treatments, however, with their emphasis on understanding and thinking, do not offer a quick fix, and demand painstaking work from both patient and therapist.

I intended that this book should give a clear outline of the rationale for dynamic psychotherapy and its place in psychiatry and in medical practice. I hope trainees and students find it useful.

Recommended further reading

This is a list of books that will be useful to postgraduates who want to or need to do further reading on dynamic psychotherapy, or to undergraduates who are particularly interested. They have been selected as especially well written, though some make quite demanding reading.

Bateman A and Holmes J (1995) *Introduction to Psychoanalysis.* **Routledge, London, p. 289.**
A clearly written and accessible overview of psychoanalytic theory and its place in psychiatric practice. Enlivened by many clinical vignettes. This book gives a good outline of the contributions of major theorists. Suitable for all postgraduate trainees in psychiatry and psychiatric nursing, and interested GP trainees and undergraduates.

Kandel ER, Schwartz JH and Jessell TM (1995) *Essentials of Neural Science and Behavior.* **Appleton & Lange, Stamford, CT, p. 741.**
An excellent textbook of neurobiology written by authors who are interested in the neural activity relating to behaviour and who respect the place of psychotherapy in the treatment of behavioural problems. Enthralling clinical histories in some chapters make it an easier than expected read. Suitable for both undergraduates and postgraduates.

Bolton D and Hill J (1996) *Mind, Meaning and Mental Disorder: the nature of causal explanation in psychology and psychiatry.* **Oxford University Press, Oxford, p. 386.**
Philosophy of mind for people working in the field of mental health. This is not a book to pass exams, but to make us examine our assumptions about what the mind is and how it works. Well written, some of it accessible and some rather more taxing. Truly exciting if you have time and motivation to work at it.

Skinner R and Cleese J (1983) *Families and How to Survive Them.* **Methuen, London.**
An entertainment, but with good educational content. Outlines the theory behind family function and dysfunction. Useful for students at any level and an easy read.

Caper R (1992) *Immaterial Facts. Freud's discovery of psychic reality and Klein's development of his work.* **Aronson, New Jersey.**
Clear and popular with postgraduates.

Fancher ER (1973) *Psychoanalytic Psychology: the development of Freud's thought.* **WW Norton and Company, London, p. 241.**
A useful summary of Freud's major theoretical ideas. For postgraduates interested in Freud and psychoanalysis.

Appendix 1
Freud: biographical details

Sigmund Freud 1856–1939

Sigmund Freud was born in what is now Czechoslovakia, but moved as a small child to Vienna, where he spent most of his life. He qualified as a doctor and worked first as a neurophysiologist and then as a neurologist before giving up his orthodox medical career to pursue his interest in exploring the effect of the mind on human behaviour. He was the founder of psychoanalysis and saw it both as a way of studying mental processes and as a mode of treatment.

He published a large number of books and papers of which the most famous include:

- *The Interpretation of Dreams* (1900)

- *The Psychopathology of Everyday Life* (1901)

- *Three Essays on Sexuality* (1905)

and the paper *Mourning and melancholia* (1917), a classic essay on the relationship between loss and depression.

As a Jew, Freud had to leave Vienna in 1938, allowed by the Nazis to escape with his family only because of his prestige. His four sisters died in Auschwitz. Freud himself died in London a year later.

The house in north London which was briefly his home is now the Freud Museum and his consulting room there can be seen as it was during his days as a practitioner in Vienna.

The Freud Museum, 20 Maresfield Gardens, London NW3.

Appendix 2
Some important names in dynamic psychotherapy

This is a short and selective list of some of the most influential writers since Freud's time. The ideas of Freud himself and those of Melanie Klein have already been discussed in more detail. The books mentioned here are more demanding than other recommended texts.

Michael Balint 1896–1970

Michael Balint came to Manchester from Budapest in 1939. He is best remembered outside psychoanalytic circles for his enthusiasm for stimulating understanding of psychodynamic principles among non-specialists, in particular GPs. Similar clinical discussion groups for exploring the dynamics of non-psychotherapy cases are still called 'Balint groups'.

Further reading

Balint M (1957) *The Doctor, His Patient and The Illness*. Pitman, London.

Wilfred Bion 1897–1979

Bion was born of English parents in India. He was educated in England, where he practised for most of his life, finally moving to the USA for his last 10 years. His experiences in the army in the Second World War led to an interest in group processes. His thinking as a psychoanalyst was very influenced by Melanie Klein. He further developed her work on projective identification and introduced the notion of the analyst who acts as a container for the patient's projections, by accepting them without excessive anxiety and without retaliating. The experience of having his difficult projected feelings calmly accepted allows the patient to feel less anxious about the feelings, so that they can be acknowledged and dealt with rather than compulsively projected.

Further reading

Bion WR (1961) *Experiences in Groups*. Tavistock, London.
Bion WR (1962) *Learning from Experience*. Heinemann Medical Books, London. Reprinted by Karnac Books, London (1984).

John Bowlby 1907–1990

John Bowlby's work as a psychoanalyst and child psychiatrist was influenced by his interest in animal behaviour. He considered that much could be learned about early human development by using systematic observation. His interest in the effects of separation on children led to the development of his theory of the place of attachment in human behaviour.

Further reading

The trilogy:
Bowlby J (1969) *Attachment and Loss Vol 1: Attachment*. Hogarth Press, London.

Bowlby J (1973) *Attachment and Loss Vol 2: Separation*. Hogarth Press, London.

Bowlby J (1980) *Attachment and Loss Vol 3: Loss*. Hogarth Press, London.

Erik Erikson 1902–1994

Erik Erikson was born in Germany of Danish parents and spent his working life first in the USA and later in London. He is well known for his ideas on child development, and emphasised the importance of the social factors in the development of the person. Erikson's best remembered contribution to psychodynamic thought was his notion that we progress through eight life stages which have to be negotiated: the stages of basic trust vs. basic mistrust; autonomy vs. shame and doubt; initiative vs. guilt; industry vs. inferiority; identity vs. role confusion; intimacy vs. isolation; generativity vs. stagnation; and finally ego integrity vs. despair.

Further reading

Erikson E (1977) *Childhood and Society*. WW Norton, New York.

Michael Foulkes 1898–1976

Michael Foulkes trained in medicine and psychoanalysis in Germany and moved to London in 1933. During the Second World War he was one of the army psychiatrists who worked in Northfield Military Hospital which was run for a time on therapeutic community lines, stimulating his interest in group work as a model of treatment. On returning to civilian life he continued to write about group methods and was the founder of group analysis.

Further reading

Foulkes M (1948) *Introduction to Group Psychotherapy: studies in the social integration of individuals and groups.* Heinemann, London. Reprinted by Karnac Books (1983).

Foulkes M and Anthony EJ (1957) *Group Psychotherapy: the psycho-analytic approach.* Penguin, Harmondsworth. Revised in 1973.

Anna Freud 1895–1982

Anna Freud, Sigmund Freud's youngest child, extended the work of her father to develop techniques of psychoanalysis with children. She also wrote about psychological mechanisms of defence. Having left Vienna for London with her parents in 1938, she established the Hampstead Nursery for refugee children during the Second World War. This later became a clinic for child psychotherapy.

Further reading

Freud A (1966) *Normality and Pathology in Childhood.* Hogarth Press, London. Revised and reprinted by Karnac Books, London (1980).

Heinz Hartmann 1894–1970

Heinz Hartmann was the founder of the ego psychology school of psychoanalysis which developed directly from the writings of Sigmund Freud and Anna Freud and has flourished in the USA. Hartmann questioned Freud's view of the ego as simply the mediator between the id and the outside world, and in 1939 wrote a mono-graph emphasising the autonomy of the ego and its capacity to operate at least in part free from conflict.

Further reading

Hartmann H (1939) *Ego Psychology and the Problem of Adaptation.* Imago, London.

Carl Gustav Jung 1875–1961

Carl Jung was the son of a Swiss Christian pastor. Jung and Freud were close collaborators in the early days of psychoanalysis but their later differences over theoretical points led to Jung's leaving the psychoanalytic movement in 1913. Jung subsequently described his ideas as analytic psychology. Jung was interested in the spiritual aspects of human experience and was particularly intrigued by the place of symbolism in the mind. He postulated that humans have universal symbols, and these ideas led to the development of his concepts of the collective unconscious and archetypes.

Further reading

Jung CG (1963) (ed A Jaffe) *Memories, Dreams, Reflections.* Collins, Routledge and Kegan Paul, London.
Jung CG (1968) *Analytical Psychology: its theory and practice.* Routledge and Kegan Paul, London.

Otto Kernberg 1928–

Kernberg is a contemporary American psychoanalyst who has written extensively about borderline and narcissistic psychopathology and its treatment. Although he recognises the contribution of environmental failure, his approach is different from Kohut's in the place he gives to innate aggression. Like Melanie Klein, Kernberg believes that some individuals are inherently vulnerable to excessive feelings of aggression which will increase their use of splitting as a mechanism to deal with developmental tasks and thus be a contributory factor in the development of borderline pathology. He suggests modification of the analytic approach in the treatment of people suffering from severe borderline pathology.

Further reading

Kernberg O (1975) *Borderline Conditions and Pathological Narcissism*. Aronson, New York.

Heinz Kohut 1913–1981

Kohut was an American psychoanalyst whose name is associated with self-psychology. He postulated the central place in development of what he called a self-object, which is his term for a person who provides the empathic responses which confirm the child's state of mind and who thus promotes maturation. Kohut considered many psychological problems to have been caused by environmental failure in early life and thought that excessive aggressive feelings were mainly secondary to such experiences. He emphasised the importance of empathy more than interpretation in psychoanalytic treatments, particularly of patients with predominantly borderline or narcissistic pathology. Kohut believed that patients with narcissistic pathology have a fragile sense of self and precarious self-esteem, and need the real and repeated experience of feeling understood in the therapy to build a more solid sense of self able to withstand the vicissitudes of everyday life.

Further reading

Kohut H (1971) *The Analysis of the Self*. Hogarth, London.

Donald Winnicott 1896–1971

Donald Winnicott was a paediatrician and psychoanalyst who worked in London. He had a particular interest in the early mother–infant relationship. He coined the phrase the 'good enough mother', to describe a mother who gives her child a quality of care 'good enough' to promote healthy development. He was especially interested in how the child learns to distinguish his mental images or fantasy from the real external world, and emphasised the importance of the child's learning to accept that his world was not under his own control. Winnicott is well known for his ideas on the essential place of play in the child's development and of the use of a transitional object as a stepping stone in learning to give up the fantasied control of an object or person.

Further reading

Winnicott DW (1971) *Playing and Reality*. Tavistock, London.
Winnicott DW (1958) Hate in the countertransference. In: *Through Paediatrics to Psycho-Analysis*, pp. 194–203. Tavistock, London. Reprinted by Hogarth, London (1975).
Winnicott DW (1958) Psychoses and child care. In: *Through Paediatrics to Psycho-Analysis*, pp. 219–28. Tavistock, London. Reprinted by Hogarth, London (1975).
Winnicott DW (1958) Transitional objects and transitional phenomena. In: *Through Paediatrics to Psycho-Analysis*, pp. 229–42. Tavistock, London. Reprinted by Hogarth, London (1975).

Appendix 3
Writing a dynamic formulation in psychiatry

As part of their training in psychiatry, junior doctors are required to make a dynamic formulation after taking a history from patients. This skill is a requirement in the examination for membership of the Royal College of Psychiatrists.

When a clinician who does not know the patient well is writing a dynamic formulation, it should be kept simple. An initial formulation is tentative. No one can really understand the dynamics of the patient's problem after a single interview, so at this stage any formulation is a working hypothesis, based on limited information.

A psychodynamic formulation is looking at psychological organisation. The formulation seeks to identify the meaning in the person's symptoms or behaviour. Why is this person having this symptom or why is he behaving in a particular way. We are trying to understand the person's internal (mental) model of himself and others and thus his conscious and unconscious expectations of his world.

- Are there any patterns in relationships or symptoms which will give a clue to there being a working model?

- Are there any obvious identifications with people in his earlier life, such as a parent?

- Can we infer any beliefs or assumptions which will make sense of or give meaning to the symptoms?

- Does he seem to use particular defence mechanisms to relate to others or to deal with stress?

One way to organise the dynamic formulation is to use the same structure as a psychiatric evaluation.

- What are the precipitating factors? What do these mean for this person?

- What are the predisposing factors? What do these mean for this person?

- What are the maintaining factors? What do these mean for this person?

Example

Paula was referred to a psychiatrist by her GP after failing to respond to a course of antidepressants. She had a baby six months ago and has felt depressed almost from the time of her son's birth. She feels constantly 'down' throughout the day and has little energy or interest in anything. She cries over trivia and is irritable with her husband, though not with the baby. Her appetite is normal and her sleep still disturbed by night feeds.

She has been married for four years. Her husband, Sam, was invited to attend the consultation but she tells you that he was too busy to take time off work. Mark is her first child. She worked as a junior manager in a large store, but decided not to return to work at the end of her maternity leave. She is not especially close to her parents who live in the north of England, about a five-hour journey away, though her mother phones regularly.

Precipitating factor: The obvious precipitating factor was the birth of the baby. What did this mean for Paula? She has become a mother. This suggests that she is likely to be at least in some ways identified with her own mother. She may also identify with her baby and his needs. The story has given some clues and indications about further information to get from Paula.

She is the eldest of three children and remembers what she calls a 'normal' childhood. Asked more specifically, she remembers that her parents split up after prolonged quarrelling lasting for several months when she was about six. This ended in her father leaving home to live with someone else. He kept in touch for a year or two but gradually lost contact with the children. She had felt she was his favourite and missed him. He now sends Christmas cards but does not remember her birthday which she still minds about. Her mother remarried three years later, but the marriage lasted only two years.

Predisposing factor: We can see a pattern here of fathers who are not there for their children. This raises the question of whether this experience is perhaps being repeated in Paula's relationship with her husband who is now also a father.

On being asked specifically why her husband did not come to the consultation Paula admits that she told him not to bother, that it was her problem and she would sort it out herself. She says they were very close until the pregnancy, but she now feels upset when he works late and feels that all the responsibility for the baby is falling on her shoulders. She enjoys looking after the baby but she is tired and not interested in sex and worries that Sam will soon lose interest and look elsewhere.

It looks as though the main problem may not be the marriage itself but Paula's expectation that it is inevitably going to go wrong.

Are there other issues which make the situation worse or which maintain the problems?

Paula has few friends locally, as she and Sam moved to the area when she became pregnant. She decided not to go back to work because she felt that the baby needed full-time care. She was in two minds about this because she enjoyed her work and the stimulation of her colleagues, but on the other hand she was determined to make a secure home for her baby. Because they are now short of money, Sam has taken on extra work. Paula worked full time until late in her pregnancy and has not yet made friends locally. She knows she should make an effort to join a mother and baby group but does not have her usual confidence. She gets lonely and feels increasingly unattractive and unlikeable.

Maintaining factors: Paula's isolation has reinforced her sense of low self-esteem and image of herself as unlikeable and incompetent. She and Sam appear to have made decisions which are rational on the surface, but which have partly unconscious determinants and whose consequences further undermine their relationship.

Formulation

It appears that the birth of her baby has revived Paula's feelings about the loss of her father. She is identified both with her mother, who could not hold on to her husband, and with the baby, whose father is not there for him. There is no objective evidence that her husband is neglecting her or the baby, but she expects him to lose interest and defensively pushes him away, for example by excluding him from the consultation. Her decision to give up work seems to have been partly coloured by her wish to give her baby more security than she felt she had as a child, and this is reinforced by her assumption that fathers cannot be relied on. She did not prepare for being full time at home in terms of arranging social contacts, so has become rather isolated. This has worsened her feeling of loneliness and lowered her self-esteem even further.

Appendix 4
Learning objectives
for undergraduates

Theory

By the end of their psychiatry firm students should be able to:

- define the term 'mental representation', explain how we acquire mental representations and explain how this is related to a person's expectations of the world

- give a definition of psychotherapy

- list the psychotherapies usually available in the NHS and describe each in 50–100 words

- give a list of the factors which Jerome Frank said characterise all psychotherapies

- explain the difference between cognitive therapy and psycho-dynamic therapy, and between psychodynamic therapy and counselling

- explain what we mean by the unconscious mind and the concept of conflict

- describe the four main points of attachment theory
- outline the implications of infant security and in security for later development.

Practice

- list the diagnostic categories which are treated in psychodynamic psychotherapy
- list the characteristics of patients who are likely to benefit from dynamic psychotherapy
- outline the aims of dynamic psychotherapy
- describe the importance of the setting, boundaries and rules
- describe what the therapist actually does, e.g. listening, encouraging, acknowledging, interpreting, etc.
- define the following: transference, countertransference, repetition compulsion, acting out
- describe group psychotherapy: how it is structured, what factors may be helpful, what patients are likely to benefit.

Further reading for those who teach basic psychotherapy

Hughes P and Gibson C (1996a) Meeting the challenge. Teaching psychotherapy to medical students, Part I: content and relevance. *Psychoanalytic Psychotherapy*. **Feb**: 1–11.

Hughes P and Gibson C (1996b) Meeting the challenge. Teaching psychotherapy to medical students, Part II: style and delivery. *Psychoanalytic Psychotherapy*. **Feb**: 13–26.

Appendix 5
Registration of psychotherapists

British Confederation of Psychotherapists
37 Mapesbury Road
London NW2 4HJ

United Kingdom Conference on Psychotherapy
167–169 Great Portland Street
London W1N 5FB

Index